I0829334

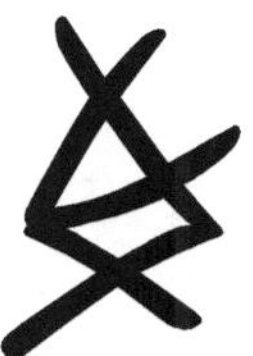

Dream Thin

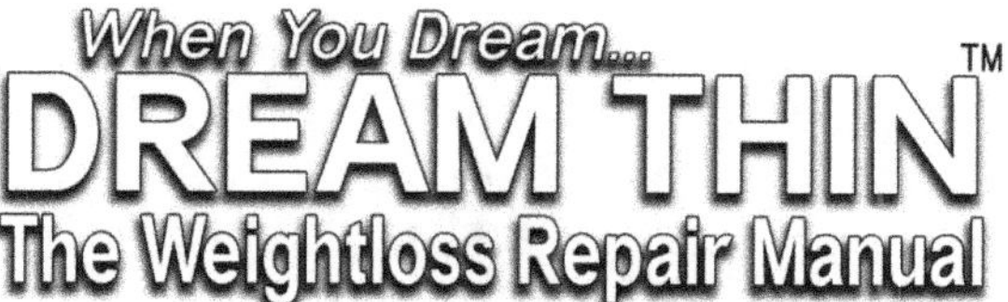

R Lindemann

Aleph Publications
Wisconsin, USA

Dream Thin
The Weightloss Repair Manual - Lose Weight While Sleeping

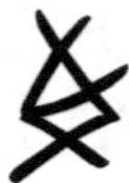

Aleph Publications
Manitowoc, WI

Paperback Edition
ISBN13: 978-1-956814-22-4

35 34 33 32 31 30 29 28 27 26   3 4 5 6 7

Disclaimer

All information, views, thoughts, and opinions expressed herein are those of the author(s) and are being presented only for your consideration and should not be interpreted as advice to take any action. Any action you take with regard to implementing or not implementing the information, views, thoughts, and opinions contained within this published work is your own responsibility. Author(s), publisher(s), and distributor(s) of this work are not liable for your choices or actions.

Anyone, especially those who have been victim of misdirected explanation and understanding, may be best served seeking wise counsel before deciding to implement any information, views, thoughts, opinions, or anything else that is offered for your consideration in this work. All information, views, thoughts, and opinions in this work are not advice, directive, recommendation, counsel, or any other indication for anyone to take any action. All information, views, thoughts, and opinions offered herein are offered only as suggestions for your personal consideration, which is done of your own free will. Your life is your own responsibility; use it wisely.

Any use of trade names or mention of commercial sources is for informational purposes only and does not imply endorsement or affiliation.

Consult with your Nutritionist-Physician before making any changes in your eating or exercise levels and considering anything else offered in the information contained herein.

Dedication

This book is dedicated to all who have struggled to lose weight and who feel like they have lost that battle. Know that it is possible to overcome weight loss obstacles and win your weight-war by being a victorious you!

Whether you have struggled in the past, or if you are now struggling, and for anyone who will struggle in the future, this book is dedicated to you. This book is here that you may know that others understand your plight, and it is also here to offer consolation and considerations. Understanding this information may ease those troubles and assist in your understanding to help you be victorious in your own personal weight loss war. You will win it if you truly want it!

Contents

Chapter 1
Conceive the Right Ideas 1
This Book is Only for Those Who Are Serious About Losing Weight 3
Terminology Basics 3
Basic Calories Per Gram 6
Key Foods Calories Per Ounce 7
Volume versus Weight 7
The Butter Factor 8
What DreamThin Isn't 9
What DreamThin Is 9

Chapter 2
Your Healthy Existence 11
High Fats & Cholesterol 11
Your Physical Discomfort 12
Suck It In or Stretch It Out 13
Taking Supplements 16
Bone and Joint Supplements 17
Healthy Dead People 19
Self-Control is what Allows You to Succeed 20

Chapter 3
Working Towards a Higher State of Being 23
Your Weight Highs and the Discouragement of the Lows 24
We Won't Hear the Good with the Bad 31
Avoiding the Wrong Action When We Feel Down 33
Avoiding the Wrong Action When We Feel Good 33
Will I Ever Feel Attractive Again? 34
Riding High 35

Chapter 4
The Way Things Happen 37
I was Once Young and Fit 37
How Did I Get So Fat 38
Changes in Our Eating Habits over the Years 39
Current Habits 39
How Air-conditioning Made Us Fat 42
Changes in Food over the Years 44

Chapter 5
Breath of Silent Techniques 49
I Just Want to Lose Weight... Now! 49
What to Do 51
Clearing of the System 52
Doing It Right 54
Importance of Accuracy 55
How to Stay in Control... Forever 56
Be Constant and Be Patient 57

Chapter 6
Adding Up the Costs 59
Medical Healthcare Costs of Being Fat 60
Health Costs of Being Fat 61
Strictly Financial Aspects of Being Fat 63

Become Aware 64
Get that Control Back 66
Dream Dollars 68
Part 1–Calculating DreamThin Dollars 69
Part 2–Be Accurate 74
Part 3-Record it All 78
Part 4–Patience 80
Part 5–Relax and Enjoy Life 82
Why It is Worth It? 82
To DreamThin 83

Chapter 7
Divide and Multiply Your Biology 87
Food is Not Evil, Food is a Gift ! 89
Fat ! Is it a Gift or is it Torture? 91
What and Why and How that Affects You 93
I Want to Gain Weight, Not Lose Weight 93
Our Bodies Will Seek Needed Nutrients 95
How Much Should I Eat? 95

Chapter 8
Things to Know About Your Body 97
Health of a Nation 99
The Family Disease Lie 101
The Genetic Lie 102
Family Habits that Cause Our Health Problems 103
Dangers of Being Overweight 105

Chapter 9
Health and Mental Protections 107
Keeping Heathy Kidneys 108
Keeping a Healthy Liver 109
Keeping a Healthy Pancreas 110
Keep that Heart Pumping 111
The DreamThin Approach 111
Ease of DreamThin 112
How to Use DreamThin Checkbook Journal Pages 112
Logging It 113
Your Debt and DreamThin Dollars 113

Chapter 10
Be Committed 115
Movement Matters 116
Exercise 117
Exercise Is a Bonus 118
The Most Effective Way to Exercise 118
Work It Through Your Body 120
Different Kinds of Exercise 120
What is Right for You 121
Main Exercise Considerations 121

Chapter 11
You Receive what You Eat 123
Hunger 123
Mining for Food 124
Eat Balanced Meals 126

Understanding What to Eat ... 127
Understanding How to Eat ... 128
Understand When to Eat ... 130

Chapter 12
Your Guide to Success ... 133
Real Life is Not Soundbites from Commercials ... 134
Battle of College Obesity ... 135
Beware of Bad Information ... 136
Be Knowledgeable and Understand ... 137
The Good News ... 138
Why DreamThin Works ... 139
Food Rule of Thumb ... 142
Exercise Rule of Thumb ... 144
Handy Measure Volume Conversion ... 146

Chapter 13
There Are Many ... 149
Pharma Ads ... 150
Health Insurance ... 151
Arthritis ... 153
Back Problems ... 153
Bones and Joints ... 154
Cancers ... 154
Coronary Artery Disease ... 155
Type-Two Diabetes ... 155
Gallstones ... 155
High Blood Pressure ... 156
Indigestion & Acid Reflux ... 156
Kidney Disease ... 157
Liver Disease ... 158
Pancreas Disease ... 158
Sleep Apnea ... 159
Stroke ... 159

Chapter 14
The Living Body Machine ... 161
The Dashboard of Your Body ... 162
Women Are Different Than Men, Period ... 163
Heat Up During Storage or Burning ... 164

Chapter 15
Details Everyone Should Agree On ... 167
Health Vs Fat Weight Loss ... 168
Fat Thin People ... 169
Your System, Less In, Less Out ... 171
Getting It to Pass Through Your System ... 172
How Long Will It Take to Lose this Fat-Weight? ... 173
Your Equilibrium ... 174
Technical Tidbit ... 174
Ask Your Doctor before Making Changes in Life Habits ... 175
Can I Really Lose Weight While I Sleep? ... 176

Chapter 16
Seeing Through the Lies ... 177
A Ridiculous Notion ... 177

The Food Police 178
Their Agenda 186
Dangers of Extremism 187
Do Not Make Food Out to Be Evil 187
All Food is Good 187

Chapter 17
Sharing Your Experience 189
Social Problems 189
Fear of Your Past 190
Using Your Past 190
Master Your Past 191
In a Perfect World 191
Be a Part of the Solution 192

Chapter 18
Our Desires 193
Can Someone Be Too Thin? 194
People Tell You to Eat More, But... 195
Cut Soda and Diet Soda 196
Don't Use Food as a Weapon Against Yourself 198
Don't Use Food as a Comfort Item 199
Need for Fat 199

Chapter 19
It Starts in Your Head and It Stays There 201
Accepting the Brutal Facts 201
Honesty 202
I Can't Do It 202
Don't Allow Other People to Crush Your Dreams 203
It is Your Life 204
With God as My Witness I'll Never Be Fat Again 205
Getting a True View of a Week's Portions 205

Chapter 20
An Example 207
Hey Fatty 208
What's In a Mirror 208
What You See You Will Be 210
What is a Calorie 211
The Important Math 211
A Kitchen Survey 213
Sorting Out Too Much Information 213

Chapter 21
It's Not My Fault 215
It's always someone else's fault 215
Us Against Them 216
Don't Go There 216
Eat It All 217

Chapter 22
Question It 219
How do you ask a question? 219
You Must Allow Yourself to Ask 220
Ask Yourself How 220
Ask Yourself Why 220

Chapter 23
A Matter of Choice 223
Surviving the Family Years 223
The Cost of Beauty 224
Depression 225
Female Negativity, But Men Do It Too 226
Who Are My Friends and Who Are My Enemies? 227
Accept It and Speak It 228

Chapter 24
Your Promise of Success 229
Why Lose Weight? 229
Put It All On the Table and Be Honest 230
Getting It Right 231
Making It Permanent 231
It's All About Balance 232
Your DreamThin Oath 233
Journal Pages 237

Acknowledgements

With every book I have written there has been a great team of support around me. Despite the delays and difficulties that come with composing a book like this one, they have held fast to their belief in what I was working towards. They have stood steadfast in the belief that at some point all of the work would come to fruition and finally be available to those who need and want the information to improve their circumstances and their lives. Thank you all for your support and assistance! It will not be forgotten.

Introduction

The philosophy behind DreamThin is simple, true, and very possible to achieve by anyone who seeks a better, healthier life. I suppose any weight-loss program will have several steps you must follow to achieve *the holy grail of health*—A perfect weight!

Don't think of properly done weight loss as some tedious seven-step-program. True and lasting weight loss will come only in understanding a set of very basic principles that we should all abide by every moment of every day of our lives, including during our sleep time. Weight loss doesn't start with what you choose to put in your mouth, but rather what you choose to put in your head. That is to say, what you put in your mind.

Nearly all of us have witnessed scores of people spending hundreds and even thousands of dollars on seven-step books and memberships and special foods, only to watch most of those people gain weight during nearly the entire process. Or they lost some weight only to gain even back more than they lost to begin with.

How is it possible that eating low-fat foods, drinking only water and diet drinks, and even exercising ends in someone getting bigger, rather than smaller? I feel quite confident in assuming that if this did not happen to you, then you likely know others and have observed this yourself while watching them struggle, ultimately losing their battle with fat.

Yes, it can be done, and it will be done by anyone who wants it. You don't even have to want it all that bad, because you can easily do it when you get your thinking right. And then it miraculously occurs on its own with little or no effort by you.

There are no hard and fast rules to follow to get the weight off when living DreamThin. Just live the DreamThin Philosophy and you are likely to win your own battle against excessive fat in all of the wrong places. It really is very simple, and alas, "simple" does not extract massive amounts of money from your pockets to pad the pockets of others as we buy program after program and meal after meal only to get even fatter and fear the scale the evermore. When reading books having to do with anything health related, it is important that you read and understand the entire book and consult with your physician *before* making any changes.

This book cuts through the fog of lies and reveals the many not-so-secret "secrets" of those who seem to stay naturally fit without even trying. And you can do it too!

Chapter 1

Conceive the Right Ideas

Are you tired of exercising for a week or two only to find that you actually gained the weight that you intended to lose? Angry that the scale keeps taunting you? Are you fed up with your mirror mocking you every time you set foot in front of it? Sick of regularly upsizing your clothes? If so then you have come to the right place.

But if you're offended at the word "fat" in reference to a person being overweight, then this book is probably not for you. *Overweight* says nothing about *why* we are overweight, but "fat" on the other hand, is very specific. *Fat* is not what you are, but rather it is what you want to rid yourself of. If you get angry when someone makes a comment that you're fat, then you probably believe that ***you are*** fat, rather than that *you **have** fat* on you. And there is an important distinction between those two views.

The DreamThin Philosophy is about getting your thinking right above all else. Sure, this book will take you through some more specific details you need to know that we are often not told, but the ideas that have been planted in your head by profiteering entities might not always be helpful to you; however, they are very helpful to them. Getting the right ideas into your head with firm understanding of the *hows* and *whys* of fat-weight loss will elevate your mind in ways you have likely never imagined.

It starts with what you conceive in your mind. If your mind has been seeded with the seeds of weeds, then weeds are what your life will produce. This of course goes beyond the weight loss topic, but we'll stick to the topic at hand because that is why you are reading this book. A great deal of what you have learned, or what you might think you have learned, is likely wrong with regard to weight loss. And beyond all other efforts it should now be your quest for your mind to be re-conceived regarding weight loss.

To make the point a bit more clear, you, and you alone, are responsible for what you choose to believe and/or follow. The information, views, thoughts, and opinions in this book are not advice, directive, recommendation, counsel, or any other indication for you to take any action. It is all offered only as *suggestions* for you to *consider* and is not for you to specifically follow in some foolish blind manner. If you want to succeed in permanently losing the unwanted pounds, you then need to be able to understand how to properly deal with the information you receive. Ask yourself: Is it good information? Or is it bad information? Will it harm me? Or will it assist in my goal? And does it unnecessarily pad the pockets of the profiteers without actually helping me?

Don't get me wrong, there are many programs out there that are well worth the value, but too often we buy programs, machines, or food and nutrient regiments that cost us much money and time, but gain us little. If you're not going to use it or follow it properly, then why waste your hard-earned cash on it?

In this book we get to the core of why we have gained the weight. For most people the "*why*" is likely not what they have thought in the past. After reading this book, most people have an entirely new understanding, thus making it far easier to master the problem of excess fat. If you're the type to defend being overweight as some type of badge of honor while saying "big is beautiful" then you could possibly find this book, or for that matter, any book that discusses getting to a "healthy weight" as offensive. So get ready, because sometimes removing the sliver from your foot hurts–a lot! DreamThin was not written to pad or protect anyone's fragile ego or emotions. DreamThin is written to cut to the core of the problem and then extract and remove the infected thoughts and replace them with good and proper thoughts that will remove and heal the problem.

This Book is Only for Those Who Are Serious About Losing Weight

If you're the type who always complains about your weight but refuses to take initiative, then this book can likely help you. But if any person is too stubborn to deal with the details, then it's hard to tell what will become of their excess fat after they read this book and work to adjust the things they have learned about weight loss throughout their life. If you're not serious about dealing with the problem, then you will very likely fail. However, if you want to move on with your life and be more healthy and fit, while looking good at the same time, then your chances of success have increased exponentially.

The problem that many of us have regarding our weight, exercising, and our food, comes in our misunderstanding a few basic points that explain a lot about *us* and our understanding.

Terminology Basics

When needed, additional terminology will be mentioned throughout, but let's get a few of the key items laid bare so that they are more clear to everyone. The first thing about terminology that we must all grasp is that pop-culture terms are generally meaningless because their meanings change more rapidly than does the wind.

Due to pop-culture, one person will think that the term "thin" means anorexic-like, where another person will see the term as being in perfect shape and ***not*** anorexic-like. We also have the term "skinny" which has similar confusion as does "thin", one person sees "skinny" as being perfectly fit and healthy, but they see "thin" as anorexic; where on the other hand, another person will see those two words as the complete opposite of that. Then we have the term "curvy", which for many people has come to be associated with a more gentle way of saying someone is fat. But many others see "curvy" as a description of a woman who has a smaller waist and wider hips and somewhat larger breast size and yet is *not* at all overweight or fat.

The reason that these terms are not consistent in each person's understanding of them is because they are arbitrary terms that do not have specific parameters. *Thin*, *skinny*, and *curvy* are all relative terms that each one of us can see in our own way as we assign our own values to them. This is neither good nor bad but does confuse things. In our social media world, everyone is eager to offer their incorrect and insensitive opinions, and they get much attention when using these sorts of relative terms. When their followers or other vulnerable people read these posts that are festering with cruelty, they then are drawn into the lies regarding the values assigned to these words that one disgruntled person posted online.

The real problem with this is that the marketers will jump on any opportunity to exploit any word that will assist them in selling their products. This in itself is not bad or evil, but if clothing companies can make their "fat-clothes" sound more sexy or appealing by referring to them as clothes for "curvy figures" then we are more likely to purchase those clothes. When they do this then they have redefined the term "curvy" in our pop-culture-minds. The same is true of the term "skinny" as in "skinny jeans". These types of terms should be ignored because someone can speak negatively about being "curvy" and indirectly be meaning fat, so someone who is naturally curvy and is in very good physical shape will be insulted or confused with the comment, thinking that they are being criticized and are indirectly being called fat.

It is our misunderstanding of such terms that causes many of us to take on an added feeling of inadequacy. It's bad enough that our culture makes it tough to stay fit and healthy, we do not need the added feeling of insult along with it.

Adding to all of that, if one man says he prefers a "curvy woman", then he likely meant that he prefers women with a small waist and wider hips and larger breasts. But a woman who is overweight could easily take this as her curvy overweight figure is what appeals to that man, when it actually is not. The problem with this type situation is that it can give that woman the wrong impression making her think that the man is attracted to overweight women. This could cause her to think that being "curvy" in that way is more desired by him, when it is not.

When we're overweight, we are all subject to the easiest route to feel good about ourselves. If we are in some way allowed to believe that "big is beautiful", then that is likely the route we will choose–but it is probably not the healthiest route to choose. Also, terms such as "big is beautiful" more typically tend to cause us to feel *worse* about ourselves than they do to make us feel *better* about ourselves.

There are many such terms in pop-culture that have been damaging the personal perspective we each have of ourselves, and as a result, that has caused many of us to feel lowly about ourselves. We embrace terms like "big is beautiful" to make ourselves feel better, but that does nothing to assist our health or help us lose weight in any way.

In weight loss terminology, we also have the often misunderstood technical-terms such as "calorie". A calorie is actually a **kilo**calorie or *1000 calories*. But in our abbreviated society we care little about specifics and so we just use the term "calorie" instead of **kilo**calorie or *Kcal.* So, in keeping with the general popular understanding of a "calorie", we will ***not*** be calling a calorie a Kcal or a kilocalorie, instead we will stick with the word the general public is comfortable with and is used on nutritional labels—"Calorie".

When we are hooked on the incorrect ideas behind any words used here in this book or anywhere else in society, then we will certainly face problems while trying to reduce the unwanted fat on our bodies. There are far too many wrong impressions about foods and weight and fat, such as *this* food is bad for you or *that* food is bad for you; or being overweight runs in my family because it's *genetic*, etc.

Fat is *fat* and it stores in us just as it does in animals. Fat is good and we would die without it. However, as our human nature would have it, we tend to overindulge and so we end up storing fat, sometimes in unhealthily large quantities.

"Calories" in a pound of *this* or *that* might seem like a trivial matter, but understanding roughly how many calories are in a given food at a glance will help you a great deal going forward.

Following is a list of some of the key terms and their calorie value that we should all become readily familiar with so that we can improve our judgement when eating:

Basic Calories Per Gram

- Fat has 9 calories per 1 gram
- Protein has 4 calories per 1 gram
- Carbohydrates have 4 calories per 1 gram
- Dry Sugar has 4 per calories 1 gram
- Dry Flour has 4 per calories 1 gram
- 100proof/50percent Alcohol has 3 calories per 1 gram

There are about 29 $^{1/3}$ grams in 1 ounce

Key Foods Calories Per Ounce

- Cooked boneless lean meat is protein and is about 53 calories per 1 ounce by weight
- Butter is mostly fat and is roughly 210 calories per 1 ounce by weight
- Flour is a carbohydrate and is about 56 calories per 1 ounce by volume
- Sugar is a carbohydrate and is about 110 calories per 1 ounce by volume
- 100proof/50percent Alcohol has 82 calories per 1 ounce by volume

Volume versus Weight

When looking at the calorie values listed above, you might have noticed that there is a difference in the calories per ounce between flour and sugar but they are the same when measured in grams. Generally, weight is the best way to determine calorie value for ingredients, but since most recipes are based on measuring with volume, volume ounces are often used rather than weight ounces. Fluffy powdered items such as flour are much lighter in weight for a cup filled than an ingredient such as granulated sugar. And *powdered* sugar can be lighter than *granulated* sugar if it is fluffed and not packed. Make sure to understand the difference between weight ounces and volume ounces. Something such as water is mostly the same when measured in weight versus volume because water is how the ounce determinations were originally created, so they are the same.

The Butter Factor

Ah... Butter... that delicious accent to our foods! Butter is fat and it is good and healthy in reasonable quantities. Butter is about 3200 calories per pound and it is a great example for you of the size or volume of the stored fat in *your* body. Imagine if you will, your excess weight in pounds equated in butter. If you are 50 pounds overweight then picture 50 boxes of butter. *One pound boxes* mind you, not *sticks.* That is how much larger you are than you ought to be.

But on the upside of this picture, you might feel that if you ***only*** lost a pound every week or two that you have not accomplished much. Fortunately, every time you lose a pound as shown on that nasty scale, get up and actually go to the fridge and grab a one-pound box of butter or a one-pound tub of margarine. Then when you're holding it in your hands, look at it and say and realize "I am this much smaller today than I was a couple weeks ago" all while you are taking note of the physical space a one-pound box of butter takes up.

A pound is nothing small. Every pound counts, and it adds up quickly! Take two or three boxes of butter, or tubs of margarine, and look at them and then realize that your body is that much smaller when an equal weight of Body Fat is lost. Don't take this lightly–*it's a big deal to you*! You had that same amount of fat in similar size in you and it is no longer there chiming in with the scale every time you step on the scale or in front of a mirror.

What DreamThin Isn't

DreamThin is *not* drugs.

It is *not* pills or vitamins.

It is *not* exercise.

It is *not* a diet.

It is *not* dangerous surgery.

What DreamThin Is

DreamThin is a way of Life!

It is that Light of Truth you have been searching for.

It is highly effective.

It's a proper way to lose body fat-weight without surgery.

It is practical.

It is a lifestyle of understanding.

It is very accurate when you are honest about everything.

Chapter 2

Your Healthy Existence

We will discuss some of the problems with health issues in a bit. For now though, I want you to realize that if you're dead, you will no longer be here. Being fat is not what kills you, it is the side effects of being fat that steal away your life and joy. There is a lot of confusion about *what is healthy* and *what is **not** healthy* and what *will* make you fat and what *won't* make you fat

High Fats & Cholesterol

It is believed that having eating habits that are high in saturated fat can cause obesity. High levels of low-density lipoprotein or "bad" cholesterol contribute, and at the same time lower levels of high-density lipoprotein or "good" cholesterol as well. Obesity is also associated with high levels of another blood-fat called triglycerides. Over time, some of these blood fats can assist the build-up of fatty deposits in your arteries throughout your body. This is called atherosclerosis, which puts you at risk of coronary artery disease and/or stroke. It is believed that consuming these saturated fats will not in itself make you fat but it can make you unhealthy if you take in too much. If we have health issues that even thin people have, but we also have excess fat, then it tends to compound our problems and complicate things a bit more.

Your Physical Discomfort

When we gain fat-weight it typically crowds the space normally occupied by our organs, causing us a great deal of internal discomfort. So, you don't necessarily need to be big on the outside in order for this to occur on the inside, though the inner and outer fat generally do go hand in hand. Our bodies are chemical machines that will take into account our mental state. This is *not* speaking of mental instability of any sort, but rather that when we think of anything, those thoughts cause us to feel emotions and those emotions are processed by our brains and subsequently produce chemicals and certain hormones in our bodies.

These chemicals are all generally good in the proper time, place, and quantity within your body. However, what happens to us is that we overindulge in these emotions, and that is where our *stress* comes from. When we stress out, we tend to also over-indulge in food. Now add to that that the normal fat storage chemistry in our bodies activates and is assisted by the other chemistry going on from the stress, causing a somewhat targeted fat storage ability.

Sometimes that targeted fat storage is internal in our abdomen and ribcage area where things can quickly get crowded for space, causing us a great deal of discomfort and strain on the adjacent organs, lending to much discomfort and even acid reflux or indigestion. There are far too many people who can't sit comfortably because of too much fat in their abdomen and ribcage area. A person who has too much excess fat will often find that it is difficult to breathe normally due to this crowding of the organs.

While many of us have gone down this path at some point in life, it is clearly not good for our health and greatly stresses our bodies.

In addition to the internal issues that fat causes, we also have the physical and appearance discomfort of being fat on the outside. There are the little things like when rashes occur between folds of skin or from our thighs rubbing together etc. Then there are, of course, the subtle emotional issues, such as how poorly we feel about ourselves when everyone else but us can fit in the seat or through the narrow passage, and finally, we generally feel less attractive.

Suck It In or Stretch It Out

Oh the things we do to our bodies. If you have ever observed an active two-year-old at play, you will quickly realize why as we age we have a tendency to gain weight. The physical motions that most two-year-olds make keeps them in very good physical shape. This includes all parts of their bodies. If you question this, then consider trying to duplicate their movements on a similar size world scaled up to your equivalent size. When someone is only about half your height and they go up the stairs on their feet, it's like you stepping up a sixteen-inch rise in each step rather than the typical eight-inch rise. Everything is twice the size to them. They are typically in very good physical condition including their "abs" or abdominal muscles.

As we age, we begin to use our bodies differently as we reach each new stage in life, and stairs become smaller to us and easier to climb causing us to use *less* effort to do the same tasks the taller we get. Up until roughly the age sixteen to eighteen we grow, and as we grow the world becomes smaller in comparison to us making nearly every task easier, thus requiring less of our physical effort relative to our size. At about the age of six we are sat down in a desk in school and told to sit still. We do this for twelve plus years and then depending upon what we do for work as an adult, we end up sitting evermore.

When we don't use our muscles they begin to atrophy, meaning that they slowly disintegrate to a point where certain tasks are more difficult than they had been in the prime of our youth. One area on our body that gets a great deal of neglect is the abdomen. Your "ab" muscles, as a child, get a great deal of use, and in comparison to our abs as adults our abs are very strong as a child. Now add to this that we tend to eat excessively and fill our internal body cavity or abs and chest area causing our belly to protrude. When our muscles are weakened from lack of physical stress activity, those muscles will stretch, and then with each passing day we gain a tiny bit more of a hanging gut.

Women who bear children will sometimes be disadvantaged with this because carrying children will add to this, but generally women who are in their twenties, thirties, and even forties when they have children can have their abs bounce back quickly with a little effort on their part.

But for the rest of us, if we let our abdominal muscles atrophy from lack of use, we will find that it takes more effort to keep those muscles sucked in enough to avoid that hanging belly. Then when the belly hangs it allows for greater intake of foods within our entire digestive tract, including the stomach.

For anyone, mostly men, but women as well, if you don't suck in that gut you will get a paunch, or commonly referred to as a gut or beer belly. When those muscles lose strength and are being forced out from your organs, fat, and a full digestive system, then it is not just extra fat hanging off of your belly, rather it is a stretching of unused muscle from the gentle but continuous internal outward pressures.

If you relax your stomach after eating too much it pushes out as is often depicted on TV with men loosening their belts after a big holiday meal. Doing this daily leads to stretched muscle tissue, thus giving your intestines more room to expand. This leads to larger intestinal volume which only presses out with greater force as the "abs" area begins to hang over the belt. The more the abdomen pushes out, the more gravity has its way with it.

To remedy this undesired situation, people who are successful in reversing this will reduce their servings and serving sizes when eating. They get into a habit of pulling their ab muscles back to their God-given flat position. As we do this over time, we can regain much of our previous figure or physique.

For many people, addressing this problem quickly reduces their weight on the scale but not necessarily much of their fat. A typical healthy person's digestive system holds from about three to ten pounds of food and waste, but some people have been found to have more than forty pounds of food and waste in their digestive system. This is why we will lose weight, it is very fast the first couple of weeks when we start to diet, and is the largest contributor to failed diets.

When we decide to go on a diet, we will typically reduce our portions and eat less all around. As we do this, our digestive system will begin to empty out, thus giving us the appearance of rapid weight loss.

Too often we are lured by fad-diets that offer seven to fourteen pounds of weight loss in the first two weeks. If you follow their diet plan, your digestive system will empty considerably, plus you will likely lose some retained water, allowing them to accurately make such claims. But what you typically don't hear from those commercials is that the rapid weight loss will come to a screeching halt at after the first week or two when you hit the dreaded "plateau" of weight loss. And you likely haven't lost an ounce of what you actually want to lose, which is the *fat* that you so desperately want gone.

What most of us don't understand as we venture in to our diet in effort to reduce our fat weight is that, when your digestive system is full of what we have eaten and it digests that food, our body is drawing off of that for survival, and our bodies do what we tell them to with regard to our actual physical and eating actions. If we give the body excess food, then the entire chemistry of the food will be digested, and in doing so, our bodies will keep drawing out any and all components it needs, and then it either stores or passes the remainder through your system.

When your digestive system is filled, it is nearly impossible to lose fat-weight. As we diet, we quickly empty the excess material in our digestive system. And until that system is emptied to a reasonable level, we are not really going to lose any fat.

When we diet, we think we are doing really well those first two weeks, but we're really not losing fat the first week or two, instead it's generally only food being emptied from our digestive system.

Fat-weight loss doesn't start until *after* the intestine's contents are reduced to a point where the absorption of calories is less than the body's burning of calories. It is the weeks after the first two weeks when most of us think we hit our perceived "plateau" when we finally actually begin to lose fat. The slow process of fat-weight loss, disguised as a plateau, is the real weight loss part, and it takes time.

Those who are successful at weight loss either know to suck in their gut, or they suck in that gut without realizing that they are doing it. To assist in fat-weight loss it helps to suck it in and have strong abdominal muscles. Exercise is usually the best way to accomplish strengthening atrophied ab muscles.

Taking Supplements

It's always best to consult a good physician when considering dealing with a weight problem or any health problem for that matter. As you begin to alter eating habits and your digestive system becomes somewhat emptied, your body will need proper nutrition. Often when we diet, we will short our body's daily food needs to a point where our body is using more calories than it is taking in. During this time it is common that our body will be shorted some important nutrients depending upon our chosen foods. And so, depending on how long someone is going to reduce their food intake to low enough levels to actually burn off the excess fat, their Vital Aminos or *Vitamins* may also end up being shorted. So depending upon what your doctor suggests, it's helpful for some people to take multivitamin supplements during their dieting or reduction period. Check with your physician.

Bone and Joint Supplements

As we gain weight, the excess fat-weigh puts extra stress on our body. This is especially true with our bone structure and joints. The lower on our body that the joints are, then the more stress those joints will experience. Some people will swear by bone and joint supplements to help keep those joints healthy, and that is good, but it is better to not have the joint problems occur to begin with.

Our bodies are amazing machines that will generally self-repair when given the right nutrients and opportunity to have enough time to actually heal. But when we are too fat, then our joints never get the opportunity to heal due to the day-to-day abuse our excess fat-weight causes our joints. Even if you have all of the required nutrients on a regular basis, you can still damage your joints by being too heavy. Our bodies, amazing as they are, can only handle so much stress before they fatigue and eventually parts begin to fail when they are not adequately cared for.

It is easiest for our bodies to self-repair when the damage done to joints is minimal. The worse the joint damage gets, the more difficult it is for our bodies to correct that damage even if we are otherwise healthy. The sooner we address the problem with proper rest and proper nutrition, then the sooner the body can repair itself. But when we collect too great of an amount of excess fat-weight, then our joints never get a chance to heal properly because we have to walk and move around as we live our day-to-day lives. We experience this most often in knees and hips and also in joints below the knee if we are substantially over our proper, healthy weight.

Runners and extreme athletes also experience such problems, even though they are in otherwise great health. If we don't give our bodies enough time to heal then they never will. This is true with any part of the body. Make sure that you are getting enough of the proper nutrition to keep your joints healthy, and also make sure to give those joints opportunity to heal between workouts if you exercise a lot.

When you have excess fat-weight, it can be cumbersome to move about while doing common daily tasks, but when we keep moving and doing those tasks, we generally keep our bodies strong and healthy while reducing our fat-weight. Physical activity is good for our bodies especially when it requires reasonable amounts of strength to do the task at hand.

One of the reasons that children are so resilient is because their bodies get a great deal of healthy strain during normal play. As we age and reduce that sort of activity, we inadvertently reduce a certain level of the *good strain* on our muscles and bones that helps to strengthens them. When our bones are used in a safe and healthy way, they are strengthened, but when they are not used much for any sort straining activity whatsoever, then our bones tend to become less strong and more brittle as we age.

When we break a bone, the bone can heal through calcification of the fractured area. It's a sort of bone-glue that our body provides naturally, and when we properly use our bodies then our bones flex very slightly causing a healthy type of micro-fracture that causes calcification keeping the entire bone strong. But when we lack this, then the calcification slowly dissolves and our bones become more porous. As we age we typically become less active, and as the dissolution of calcium occurs in our bones and the porousness increases, our bones become lighter and weakened and thus, when we fall we break a hip that would not have broken thirty years prior from the same type of fall. This tends to be more common with older women in their sixties and seventies and beyond, which makes sense because women tend to take jobs that require less physical strain and are usually more mentally or emotionally focused. Often women work at desk jobs or care for their family or have a job that doesn't cause much physical strain on the bones. After many years of this, the bones get more porous, making them more susceptible to fracture upon impact from falling. Adding to that, our bones are also affected by our body chemistry, namely from our hormone levels.

Healthy Dead People

What is a healthy dead person? If you think about people you know who are now dead and who were health-conscious people, then you probably know someone who has died at a prematurely young age. For some reason, when we obsess about our eating habits, it tends to not go well for us, which happens all too often.

Over the years, we all have watched ads for improving our health, and some of the "healthy" people in those ads were trying to save us from the doom that they feared, but they are now dead at prematurely young ages.

It sounds awful, but it's true. There are many people, who for fear of death, set out to be "healthy" and then end up dying in their fifties, sixties, or early seventies. These people ate healthy, didn't do drugs, didn't drink much alcohol, if at all, and exercised regularly, and then died, usually from heart failure or cancer. And often those that we would assume who would have had the healthiest hearts died from complications of the heart. Can we expect this same fate if we become "healthy" too?

I believe *we can **avoid** this* when we have a healthy *attitude* about foods. It is not so much what we eat that causes our problems, but rather it is how much of what we eat and what we don't eat that kills us.

Self-Control is what Allows You to Succeed

How many times have you decided to grab a snack out of the cupboard and you opened the bag or box intending to have only a few, but then find that you have eaten the entire contents of the package–all eight servings? Too many times I suspect. The problem is that it is not necessarily always some horrible uncontrollable urge that we can't seem to tame; often it's nothing more than us not paying attention to our actions.

We might be watching a movie, and while enthralled in the plot as it thickens, we somewhat unconsciously keep shoveling chips into our mouth. Then poof! The package of chips is gone! This is a difficult thing to overcome because we don't do it as a deliberate action, we don't intend to eat the *entire* thing–but we do.

How do we become health conscious without becoming a healthy dead person? The first thing is not to obsess about your eating. No food is evil, which we will discuss later. The point is to become aware and conscious of your actions without being obsessively conscious.

Pay attention when you grab a snack, and meter out what you're going to eat. Post a note on your snack cupboard to remind you to only take ***one*** serving from the bag, and then put that serving in a bowl and leave the rest in the bag and put the bag back in the cupboard. The idea is to not to specifically do that, but rather to find ways to make yourself aware so that *you* are able to consciously stop yourself from accidentally eating too much.

If you do something like posting a note in the cupboard, you will be reminded and then think, "oh yeah, only grab one serving." This way as you watch your movie, when the snack is gone, then it's gone.

Posting the note does help in becoming more conscious of your servings, but it's when you finish your single serving that helps you to become more conscious, and it will assist in regaining your self-control. You will notice when the bowl is empty—especially if you're accustomed to eating the entire package's contents.

Self-control is a tough aspect of life because often our lack of self-control is due to stress and control issues we have to deal with in our day-to-day lives. For instance, if life seems to be beating you down and you have an inner feeling that you have no control over the tough breaks that keep hitting you nearly every day, then eating is one pleasure that is yours alone and nobody can take that pleasure away from you—except you.

Eating does bring us joy and comfort. This is not a bad thing and food should be enjoyed, but we have to work towards not enjoying too much of it during a single sitting.

Self-control is a tough thing to conquer for most of us because there are so many areas to consider, which causes us to miss the fact that we are lacking self-control. Stress causes us to lose self-control. Lack of control in one area of life can cause us to lose self-control in another area of life. And mindless oblivious eating causes us to lose our self-control in the one area we should and can have the best and easiest control of.

If someone mentions that we have no self-control, it usually makes us feel insulted or humiliated, even if it's true. But think about the words for a moment "self" and "control" separately. *Self* being you and *control* being your ability to control yourself. It sounds bad when we think "my ability to control myself", it makes it sound like we are inept, uncontrolled maniacs, but that's not really what it is. Self-control is the awareness and the ability to catch yourself doing something in a somewhat unconscious manner.

Sure, some of us will eat uncontrollably, spoonful after spoonful, feeling more guilt with each one as we shovel it into our mouth, but while that's a self-control issue, it is not what we are talking about here, and it is not the problem. The reason most people gain weight is that we lack the *conscious* ability to stop eating. We eat obliviously because it feels good and we are simply not paying attention, and therefore we lose our self-control through being *oblivious* during the act of eating. It's not that we are oblivious to life or health or eating, rather it is that we just don't give it any thought as we eat. We grab and we eat and then we fail to think about it at all as we do it. Doing the little things like posting a note helps to remind us to take less as we measure out what we take.

When we eat what we have taken, we will notice when it's gone and that makes us conscious. There is no need to have your notes be a source of humiliation. Rather, you simply are working in effort to remind yourself to consider the amount you should eat during that particular sitting.

Too often we are taught to feel humiliated or shamed by our eating habits, and for some people humiliation and shame might work to suppress their eating, but self-humiliation is generally not necessary. Simply find ways to alert yourself so that you become aware of what and how much you are grabbing when you snack, because snacking is one of the biggest reasons we gain too much fat-weight, especially when it is done at night.

Self-control is what allows you succeed and it might be better stated as self-control-awareness or awareness-of-self-control. It is the *awareness* part that gives us the control of self.

Chapter 3

Working Towards a Higher State of Being

In the last chapter we discussed the issues of stress and self-control, however, we didn't really touch on *how* those sorts of things make us feel. The way we feel is a very big part of why we eat too much. We eat when we're sad. We eat when we're happy. We eat when we're nervous. We eat when we're frustrated. We eat when we feel ashamed. We even eat when we feel ashamed about eating. We just like to eat!

Eating isn't bad, and it never will be bad. But the ***quantity*** that we eat is bad when it's too much too often, and it will always be bad when it's too much too often. Maybe "bad" is the wrong word because eating is not bad and without doing it you are guaranteed death. *Proper* eating is one of the requirements of a healthy life. It's the quantity and frequency of our eating that causes our problems, and often that is dictated by our feelings.

Our feelings can cause an avalanche of eating, and that is something that we must guard ourselves against. When we overeat we typically feel worse about ourselves, causing us to over-eat even more.

One of the first areas we should consider is that it is okay to over-eat on some occasions, provided that it won't harm you; there is no need to feel guilty about over-eating on those rare celebratory occasions. There might be certain celebrations where food will be abundant and we take in far more calories than needed. But these occasions generally only occur a few times per year. For instance, your birthday might be one of those occasions when you choose to ignore reasonable limits on eating. It's generally okay to have such occasions and there is no need to feel guilty on those occasions. But those should be somewhat rare "occasions" and *not* daily habits.

When we feel badly about ourselves we tend to eat to make ourselves feel comforted. But when we eat, we gain weight and together the extra eating and the extra weight make us feel bad all over again. It is a vicious cycle.

When you work towards a higher state of being, you do better than your best to take hold of that self-control awareness mentioned in the last chapter, and then apply it to your entire life, especially to your feelings. Our feelings, or emotions, are a slippery slope of despair for us when we let things get out of control. We all need to stay ever vigilant. Some of us can pull this off with little effort, but for most of us it's a matter of vigilance–a constant awareness without us obsessing about it.

Once we master the vigilance, then our feelings and emotions lose their power over us, allowing us to live in a higher state of being.

Your Weight Highs and the Discouragement of the Lows

There is no place that uncontrolled feelings can sabotage our fat-loss efforts more than in our own feelings of discouragement. The DreamThin Philosophy is to never give up. This applies to losing control, but here we are also thinking along the lines of discouragement when you're doing everything right while trying to lose that unwanted fat.

Anyone who has ever made any attempt to lose fat will likely be able to attest to how discouraging it is to diet and exercise for several days only to step on the scale and find that you actually weigh *more* than you did before you started. But if you are truly doing things right, then never let that discourage you!

Our bodies are incredible machines that have needs to function, and they respond both to good care and to attacks. By attacks we are not talking about anything violent, but rather food and exercise. What we eat affects our body, and our body will process what we eat in accordance with its needs based upon what we have done with regard to our physical activity. Physical activity is not only exercise; physical activity can be any activity including the lack of it, such as sleeping.

As the body adjusts for our actions, it will retain foods and liquids to suit its needs. Adding to this, the particular foods we eat will also affect what the body does with those foods.

Fat loss is the goal. When you are fat, ***weight***-loss has little to do with anything because the scale can measure both fat-weight loss and overall-weight loss. Discouragement comes when we work hard and use self-discipline and self-control and do all of the right things, but then find that we have actually gained weight. ***Do not*** let this discourage you! If you exercise vigorously for an hour you might be three pounds lighter after you finish than you were when you started–just from sweating. But if you failed to hydrate yourself properly beforehand your body is going to want to replenish the lost water that you sweated out. So, when you drink liquids the rest of the day you will likely find that you do not need to urinate as often as you normally would with the same liquid volume consumption under your normal circumstances. This can cause the scale to have higher numbers when you step on it again later that day. But don't let that discourage you, water and food retention are doing you good in this case.

Weight highs and lows will always occur, and every one of us has them. It is when we understand that our body is adjusting to the circumstances at hand that we can banish our discouragement. When working to lose fat-weight *we must be in it for the long-haul.* And as they say, "it's not a sprint, it's a marathon."

Our bodies are chemical machines, and these machines have limits. So, when you workout for an hour and are two or three pounds lighter from sweating, you have likely only burned a few hundred calories of actual energy. Those few hundred calories equate to maybe an ounce of fat, if you're lucky. And the truth of the matter is that when you're done exercising the fat is generally all still there. It tends to come off afterwards as your body rebuilds after workout. And that is one of the main points of DreamThin. You don't do real fat-weight loss during exercise, it typically happens *after* exercising depending upon how long you exercised. In fact, for many people there is no need to work out because they get plenty of exercise while working at their regular job.

The only way to really judge your weight on a day-to-day basis is to average it in five-day groups every day. To do this you record your weigh every day and then take the previous four days from the current day, add them up with the current day's weight and divide by five. This offers a more accurate weight that will likely not be quite so discouraging. And if you want to be really scientific about it, weigh yourself three times a day and average that and use that as your daily number to be added to the previous four days. The problem that we have is that fat loss is somewhat of a scientific endeavor, and most of us are not scientists. Learning to do simple averaging of your fat-weight as just mentioned will assist considerably in avoiding such discouragement.

If we are stepping onto a scale for the purpose of monitoring our fat-weight loss, a day-by-day scale reading is mostly useless. We are often told to weigh ourselves first thing in the morning, and this does help with a somewhat more stable reading, however, due to the way our body machine works, it takes more time than a single day for our body to acclimate to the given circumstances of the eating and activity actions during any one day. So, when we step on the scale only once a day and then use that number, we are not really weighing ourselves, but rather we are weighing our body's response to the previous few days.

There are just too many factors to take in to account to be able to have your daily scale reading not be frequently discouraging. Daily weight readings are frustrating and cause many people to simply give up, that is why DreamThin *Averaging* is more proper and far less discouraging. DreamThin Averaging evens out the spikes in the numbers you record which is why averaging is so important for you to do if you are watching the scale closely. It is not important to weigh yourself every day, but averaging should always be done and it should include at least the four previous recorded weights. If you are not consistent regarding the time of day during which you weigh yourself, then it will serve you better to use ten instances of weigh-in (2 per day) to average if you want to remove those discouraging spikes in your numbers.

When we get serious about losing the unwanted fat, we modify our eating and do some extra physical activities, and then for the first week or two we feel like we can conquer the world because the weight is coming off so rapidly. But when your digestive system is mostly emptied and the water retention is less, the weight loss then stops or slows down to a snail's pace in comparison because now you are finally digging into that fat you so desperately want to rid yourself of. As mentioned earlier, this is because we can really only lose about an ounce or two per day. This means that real fat-weight loss will generally only be about a pound every week or two. When you need to lose thirty, forty, fifty or more pounds, that ounce or two per day is somewhat discouraging. When the initial digestive tract content weight and water weight are gone and we hit the dreaded "plateau" where the scale won't move, that is when it's very discouraging to see the scale taunt us as we retain a bit of water, or our digestive system decides to hold onto the food a bit longer causing the scale to be up a pound or two, which seemingly defeated our last two weeks of effort.

When you are only measuring an ounce or two of real fat-weight loss every day or two, that small amount of weight gets lost in the large fluctuations that occur from retained water and food. This is why using a weight average is best. Averaging at least four to seven days is the minimum to use, but the more days, up to fifteen, that are used in your average then the more accurately it will reflect your fat-weight loss progress.

Then there is the issue of the quality of the scale. Typical bathroom scales measure in two-tenths-pound increments. Some of the better scales might use a one-tenth-pound precision. Two tenths of a pound is about three ounces, and one tenth of a pound is about an ounce and a half. So if you're doing a lot of working out and taming your eating desires, you might see a one tenth reduction every day, but on a two tenths increment scale it will take two or three days to see the change on the scale's readout. What we all also need to realize about these scales is that they are not particularly repeatably accurate.

I feel certain that most of us have stepped upon a disobedient scale multiple times to weigh ourselves to make sure that we get the lowest reading at that moment. Doing so is a clear indicator that these scales are not very repeatably accurate. So, when using these scales, weight averaging also helps to even out those fluctuating readings. There is no need to average your weight of the moment. Just step on the scale once and then use that number in your five-day average. By you understanding the issue of how our bodies and how our bathroom scales work and then averaging your seven-day weigh-in results, you will reduce your discouragement a great deal.

Never give up because you blew it one day and the scale mocks you. Just make it up the during the next day or two. DreamThin Averaging takes you through ruined days, water retention, bloating, and a full digestive system by showing you exactly where your weight really is as long you stay true to your goals. DreamThin Averaging works extremely well and is reasonably accurate when you don't lie when recording your daily weight. We all must understand how the scale can fluctuate in only a matter of hours from a multitude of reasons.

When we decide to "get fit", we cut out the junk food, including soda, and start to eat fruits and vegetables knowing we are getting all healthy. And maybe we jog or walk for an hour or so each day, and then we get on the scale and find our weight increased that week after all of that effort and sacrifice. When we cut out junk foods and caffeine, and then increase fruits and vegetables, it alters our chemistry, generally causing our water retention to increase to a healthy level. Don't let that upset you.

If you're doing things right and you're not lying to yourself about your actual food consumption and exercise amount, this is normal and it is good. Your body's cells like and need that kind of moisture. It's what makes them function better, allowing you to lose fat a little bit faster. This is your true weight and it will begin to go down slowly and steadily after a couple of weeks while your body adjusts to your new healthier habits.

We can't get ourselves caught up in the typical scenario where we decide to diet and cut our calories and lose about five pounds in just a few days and then think "wow this is great! At this rate I will have all the fat gone in only a few weeks." Very little or none of that weight reduction was actually fat-weight. It is both water weight and digestive system content weight, and *only* after we deprive our intestines of our *excess* food (energy), can we start to reduce the amount of fat on our bodies. It is difficult to lose more than a few ounces per day unless you really exercise a lot, and I mean **a lot**!

If you're inaccurate in your actions, you will fail dreaming yourself thin and fail yourself, and you will stay as you are by your own choice. But if you choose to be pure and honest and make up for "bad days" by correcting those errors, and also **over**estimate rather than **under**estimate calories consumed, then you will likely hit your goals early.

Remember, a scale is only a measuring tool. In the long term your eye in the mirror is the best judge. It takes about three weeks to start to notice the real differences, and those differences will continue till you dreamed yourself thin. When being true to your new ways, people will slowly begin with compliments or at least notice how your efforts are paying off. But this doesn't mean you're done. All too often we get a compliment and then feel that we can reward ourselves, but that is not a good idea if the reward is food or deciding that you don't need to exercise that day.

Right now, you're carrying around a lot of extra fat and that takes more energy, so in the earlier stages of fat-weight loss, the more you weigh, the more quickly the fat can come off because your muscles have a lot of extra work to do as they carry around the excess fat-weight on your body. So, we have to understand that as we get nearer to our goal, the fat weight is reduced more and more and we are no longer carrying as much fat weight, thus our *muscles* no longer have to work as hard carrying the excess fat-weight. The reduced pace of fat-weight loss might seem painfully slow, but this is normal. Happily, it does come off faster in the earlier stages with similar activity levels you might do in the later stages as you get closer to your goals.

In this section we discuss exercise and eating good foods in reasonable quantities, but the exercise is only a bonus of the DreamThin way.

There are many people who want to lose fat-weight and do, but they feel "saggy" after the weight comes off. Sure, if we stretch our skin from being overweight for too long and at too old an age, then we will often have some sagginess in our skin. But the sagginess we are referencing to here has to do with our muscles. If our muscles are not used much, then we have little muscle tone, so exercise is of great assistance in how you look after losing fat-weight to help remedy the sagginess issue.

For many women who don't want bulging muscles, stretching is a very beneficial way of toning your muscles without building them beyond the desired amount. Often mistakenly referred to as "yoga", *stretches* can do amazing work on a woman's muscles without making them look like men's muscles.

Never allow yourself to be discouraged. And always be ready to hear the good with the bad. Don't attack anyone who notices that you have gotten fatter, instead take that notice as a warning-light that it's time to take matters into your own hands and control the fat, rather than letting the fat control you. And never lash out at someone who is graciously bringing attention to your excess fat-weight.

We Won't Hear the Good with the Bad

It's interesting how when we begin to lose weight, we suck up those compliments like a brand-new vacuum cleaner. But when someone notices we have gained a bit of weight, then look out or we will bite your head off!

Why can't, or won't, we hear the good with the bad? This problem is especially bad when it comes to the ones who we claim that we "love". If a husband or wife says "dear, I am concerned about your weight gain" then look out because we are often likely to tear them to shreds with our vicious words. Some of this is also touched on in the book *Red Hot Marriage - Made in Heaven Filled with Passion and Joy*. But if they notice we have lost weight, then we take it in with a bit of arrogance. Sometimes our arrogance defeats us and we feel that since someone actually noticed all of our hard work, we then deserve to treat ourselves. So we proceed to cheat our efforts and end up seeing a spike on the scale and then we get all down and depressed about it, which is why the last section about averaging the fat-weight loss numbers on the scale is so important in order for us to avoid discouragement from our foolish behavior.

Never get angry when someone notices that you have gained weight. It's not fair to that person, especially if they truly want to help you. It is also not fair to get angry if it's true. Sure there are cruel people out there who get a rise out of taunting us about our weight, but most people are generally pretty fair in their assessments of our fat-weight appearance. When someone, even the cruel people, make comments, we should and must take it as a sign that something is not right with our weight and we must then examine our situation and decide if what they are saying is actually honest and true. We usually know this already, but the fact that they have commented on it is clear indication that it is getting out of hand. For most people, it's hard for them to work up the courage to say something about someone's weight, because they don't want to hurt our feelings or be attacked by us.

We must take the bad as graciously as we take the good, and we can be pretty sure that if we cannot find it within ourselves to do that, then our weight problem is very likely more internal or emotional than it is from our physical habits and eating, because our emotions drive those habits and eating.

If someone kindly comments on our weight gain, we should be thanking them for bringing it to our attention even though we most certainly are already aware and already feel horrible about it. But their courage in pulling us aside to kindly discuss it is a monumental undertaking on their part. And when their comments prompt us to finally take action regarding what we already knew, but were too complacent to act on, then we really owe them a bit of thanks.

So it really doesn't matter what someone notices, because we should always be grateful for the notation. If we look good, then we look good, and thank you! And if we are fat, then we are fat and thank you for making me keenly aware that this is noticed by others. Recognition of our fat by others is a painful *gift* that we must utilize as motivation to get healthy.

We cannot achieve a state of higher being when we take the wrong actions when we hear what we would like to *not* hear.

Avoiding the Wrong Action When We Feel Down

Often when we have too much fat-weight, we know it. We feel badly about ourselves and then if someone else happens to mention to us that we have gained too much fat-weight, it can really break us. This is where getting yourself into a higher state of being is really important. If we allow our hurt feelings or poor self-image to dictate our eating, exercise, and all-around motivation, then we will fail. Protect yourself from being an oversensitive jerk.

Avoid taking the wrong action when feeling down–don't succumb to the snack cupboard. There's an interesting emotional effect when you "stick to it". What tends to happen when we stick to it is that, we feel better about ourselves the next day, which serves to strengthen our resolve and makes us feel better and better each time we do so, thus helping us to defeat our desire to give up.

Avoiding the Wrong Action When We Feel Good

But let us not forget that we have this awful tendency to also take the wrong actions even when we feel good about ourselves. We get compliments or maybe had some great thing occur in our lives and we feel that we deserve a treat or an oversized meal. This is not necessarily a bad thing when done only *occasionally*. But what all too often happens is that, we do this sort of I-feel-good-so-I-deserve-a-reward thing and then the scale mocks us with that error. Then we feel down and discouraged and take the wrong action again by further proceeding to drown our sorrows in snacks and treats.

It is so very important to defeat this emotional ping-pong in order for you to rise to a higher state of being so that you can achieve your fat-weight loss goals with ease.

Will I Ever Feel Attractive Again?

Being over fat-weight can be one of the most emotionally debilitating aspects of weight gain that there is, and it seems that the heavier we are then the more it can steal away our drive to achieve a higher state of being. When our joy is robbed by fat, our only true weapon to defeat the problem is to do so with the self-control spoken of earlier.

The more fat we have, the worse it seems, but in some ways, this is not true. When we notice fat piling up, even in the earlier stages of fat gain, we still often feel less attractive, but it's easy to ignore in the early stages. Among the many reasons that it is easier to ignore is our innate ability of comparison. When we set out on our fat collection expeditions and notice that our cargo bay is beginning to fill, we tend to compare ourselves only to other people who are fatter than us. But oddly, we tend to ignore those who are fit who do not have excess fat. But the more fat we gain, then the more difficult it is to find people who are fatter to compare ourselves to in order to make ourselves feel better.

As our weight increases, we see the ill-effects on our body and then shut our eyes to the problem and tend to look to others who are larger than we are in our ill attempt to make ourselves feel better. But we don't really feel any better. In fact, deep down we all know that we are lying to ourselves to cover up the shame we feel. Then to make ourselves feel better, we do the wrong thing—we eat!

It's an intriguing thing how the moment we begin to lose fat and can notice it in the mirror or even on the scale, we suddenly begin to feel better about ourselves and more attractive again.

Yes, you will feel attractive again the moment you start to lose fat-weight and can see it on the scale or in the mirror. But we usually struggle with this because when we try to lose fat-weight, we end up only losing a little bit of overall weight, but then it comes right back because we lack understanding. Understanding the basics of how your body actually works regarding fat-weight loss will in itself help you to feel more attractive by making you feel more in control. And actually being more in control helps you to avoid becoming an emotional ping-pong ball.

Riding High

When you control your fat, you feel better because your weight and emotions are no longer controlling you. Fat stored to excess has this terrible way of beating us down. This is especially true when we are not quite understanding exactly why or how we are gaining the fat-weight.

When someone or something has control over us, it is very defeating. For instance, if we get behind on our payments or bills, we typically feel like things are out of our control because we might get calls demanding payment. Well, fat is the same. Fat is constantly reminding us that we have fallen short, and when we are not sure how this happened in the first place, it's like having lost your job and you are now unable to meet your obligations.

Our first obligation to ourselves is to take care of our own body. We all know when we have gained weight, and ignoring the situation only serves to make matters worse. But when you understand the basic functions of your body regarding fat storage and fat loss, it breaks those chains that bind and hinder you from the doing something about it. Learning the basics of the inner workings of body fat is like finding a great job that will help to easily meet those obligations mentioned in the example just given.

We can all achieve this higher state of being when we understand and take a stand against our unfair fat build up in our body. Too often we seek some sort of "fairness" in life and life should be fair, but life is *not* fair, and the sooner we learn that then the sooner we can get our footing set in such a way that it is hard to knock us down. Our first task in doing so is to decide that we have had it and that we are going to make a change. The second task is to understand everything we need to know so that we can make our plans to solve the problem quickly and safely.

Without the knowledge and understanding of the basics of fat-weight loss, most of us will continue to fail at our attempts, and each failure drives us further and further down the wrong path.

All of us can find a new power over food when we understand it and when we understand our bodies, thus allowing us to reach new goals every day and achieve that state of higher being that has been eluding far too many of us for so long.

Chapter 4

The Way Things Happen

What happened? How did this happen to me? Look at my pictures from years gone by, I was a skinny kid until...

That's right "until". Until what? Maybe we had children or had a job in the food industry, or we liked all of the options for snacks over the years. This list can go on quite a while, and we have already discussed some of these reasons or at least aspects of them, such as feelings of lost control etc.

I was Once Young and Fit

Most of us don't realize this, but many of us will gain about fifty pounds of fat-weight by the time we are about forty years old–unless we are vigilant. And vigilance comes only with knowledge and understanding. As a child, up until about the age of about twenty years old, we are generally pretty active. We're busy playing and running around, maybe as a young child at play or as an older child on sports at school. We didn't have time to be munching on snacks all the time as we do at our sedentary desk jobs where there always seems to be a snack at the ready.

To make matters worse, managers at our work places will often, out of kindness or as an incentive, bring in pizza or donuts or some other very high calorie treat to the workplace to keep us happy. And happy we are... until it begins to add up on the scale after a few years or even after only a few months.

How Did I Get So Fat

Treats in the workplace is one area that we defeat ourselves, but we also have to consider our work environment itself. I enjoy fast foods on occasion and will frequent certain establishments that serve items that I like to eat. Fast food restaurants typically have a high rate of employee turnover, but for some of those employees who stay for the long-haul, that environment can be devastating to their figure.

I have no proof if the environment contributed to their weight gain, but I noticed quite a few people who worked at these establishments for long periods who slowly gained weight, and I also noticed most of them munching a fry now and then, or sipping a soda. Later in life, I had an opportunity where I could observe some of these establishments in a more direct manner and it confirmed what I was pretty sure I noticed about some employees eating little bits on the job. This is true of both males and females, but I noticed it more with young women, probably because they tend to choose to stay in some of those jobs longer than do young men.

Our worst attempt at sabotaging our own bodies is to nibble constantly. When we are in an environment where we can sip sodas or eat a single french-fry every few minutes throughout the day, then we will certainly gain that unwanted fat-weight that we all dread.

Changes in Our Eating Habits over the Years

It is an interesting thing to watch older movies and compare them with contemporary movies. You will generally notice a considerable increase in the waistlines of the people in the newer movies compared to the older movies. Sure, some people from days gone by also had problems with excess fat, but there were a lot less people who were over fat-weight years ago than there are in our modern times. And back then, the amount over fat-weight was typically less as well. What happened to us?

Current Habits

Our societal habits have changed. Depending upon your age, you will recall how advertising and products changed since you were a child. For those born in more recent decades after the advertising changes involving technology occurred, there is little awareness that things were ever different than they are today. Our habits are typically driven by what we see and what we can do and, too often, what we can get away with. As our world changed and more moms entered the workforce, our culture slowly gravitated towards eating at fast food restaurants and ready to eat snacks.

Eating out isn't bad and should not be shamed, but the quantity of food we order is an entirely different story. If we ever want to trim the waistline, then blaming the fast food restaurants for offering us larger portions will *not* do us any good. Our habits are ***our*** habits, and while they are influenced by advertising and convenience, they are still ***our*** habits. This is where the self-control issue spoken of earlier comes into play.

For those who are too young to remember, there was a time in history that you didn't always get to choose the size of drink you wanted. The drinks where served in eight-ounce glasses filled with ice and then the drink was poured in over the ice, and you had to pay for *each* glassful. Then when the drive-thru and fast foods entered the market, choice in size of drinks became commonplace. But in those early days of fast-foods, a large drink was about the size of what a small is today, and they were *filled* with ice and then the drink was added. So a sixteen-ounce large drink had only about eight to ten ounces of liquid in it. Now move to today's drink sizes and a large is now as high as forty ounces, and sometimes even higher, plus we can request no ice. But even when we do get ice it's usually only about four or five ounces in a large drink, leaving us with thirty-five ounces to drink–that's about three cans of soda. And some of us will do this more than once a day.

And let us not forget that once upon a time, soda-pop came in eight, ten, or twelve-ounce glass bottles, or in twelve-ounce steel or aluminum cans, and then eventually sixteen-ounce glass bottles. Then as our appetite grew for larger drinks, and plastics became more common, the common drink size of twelve ounces grew to sixteen and then twenty-ounce bottles as the standard. In our modern times it is difficult to find a twelve-ounce soda in a gas station or soda machine because most of them dispense sixteen- or twenty-ounce plastic bottles.

Whose fault is this? Is it the beverage companies' fault? No, it's our own fault. Collectively, we embrace these ridiculously large drink sizes, and the manufacturers will accommodate whatever we want to buy, and they will continue to do so as long as ***we*** keep buying. Every now and then we get lucky and the manufacturers scale size down to cut costs, giving us less for the same price so that they can keep the prices more stable while staying profitable. But then we whimper and wine because "we are getting cheated" as we pile on the fat because the portions sizes are still too large for our bodies to overcome the amount of calories in each portion.

Yes, it is all our own fault and we can scream at and blame the manufacturers, stores, and fast-food chains all we want. But in the end, no amount of blame will make the truth any different and it will not reduce our unwanted fat.

Our current habits are dictated by our choices, they are not dictated by what we are offered. The offerings certainly are of no help, but it is not their fault, it is ours. Most restaurants have small drinks with lots of ice available, if only we would ask or choose that route as we fill our drink cup. They also have healthier portion sizes–if you ask. Any one of us can take advantage of these other choices whenever we choose to. It is only with our awareness of the changes that occurred in our culture that we can curb our over-indulgent desires in our future.

Here is the part of this that caught many of us off-guard: When a large soda was sixteen or twenty ounces and had lots of ice in it, we ordered a large and got eight to twelve ounces of soda, then when they introduced thirty-two ounce large soda we said "crap that's huge!", but oddly we kept accepting that larger size rather than asking for a medium or a small the next time we ordered a drink.

We have gone from consuming one hundred to one hundred-fifty calories of soda back then, to up to as high as four and even five hundred calories for a single drink at a single meal today. Our entire meal total, *including* drink, should be roughly only around five hundred calories for each meal. But, for some of us, the soda is a real problem when the drink alone rivals a normal full meal in calories. But here is the worse part; we often sip that drink all day long, and doing so will destroy **any** hopes of fat-weight loss we might dream of.

While diet soda doesn't have calories as such, don't let that fool you. Diet sodas are of little or no help when used as a replacement for our bad habits. Besides the soda, we also have to consider that there have been comparable changes surrounding the foods that are served with our oversized drinks, none of which have helped our chosen habits for the better. Additionally, the non-caloric artificial sweeteners in diet soda and other such diet drinks fool our system just enough to provoke the hormonal chemistry causing the body to prepare to store calories.

How Air-conditioning Made Us Fat

There was a time years ago, and anyone reading this won't remember it. It was the time before air conditioning. To those of you born after air conditioning in homes became commonplace, *yes*, there was a time when most homes were *not* air conditioned. That's right, when it was sweltering hot at night, we had to suffer through that heat and toss and turn trying to find a cool spot on the bed or the cool side of the pillow to feel comfortable enough to actually fall asleep. Maybe that's why we were not as fat years ago–we got so much exercise tossing and turning on hot nights that we lost weight!

On a more serious note, air conditioning is a wonder and it is a wonderful gift that keeps us all comfortable and can actually save the lives of many when the heat gets very hot. But air conditioning is also our downfall. Air conditioning on hot days makes us docile and we tend to sit inside and watch TV or play on our computer devices as we trap ourselves in our homes to stay "comfortable". This has certainly not helped any of our waistlines. The real issue regarding our seemingly unexplainable increase in waist size is not from our home air conditioning, it is from air conditioning or *refrigeration* on a much larger scale.

To start with, there was a time, believe it or not, that people did not have a refrigerator anywhere in their home, and in the early days of refrigerators they were actually ice-boxes. Meaning that in winter people would go out on the lake and cut large ice blocks from the lake-ice and then that would get stored in warehouses and covered with hay to insulate it so that it would not melt so fast. Then a delivery man would bring ice to people's homes and place it in their ice-box and that would keep their food cold.

People didn't have freezers, though some items may have frozen if close enough to the ice block. And keep in mind that these ice-boxes were really quite small compared to what we have today. They certainly didn't have running water or ice crushers built in to the door. In winter, the sunporch typically became the icebox in those days.

As refrigeration was figured out, it was first implemented in industrial settings before electric home refrigerators become common. In those early days of refrigeration, ice companies no longer had to cut ice from the lakes and store it, instead they could make ice on demand and would no longer run out of ice in the fall. This meant no more waiting until the next freeze to build up their ice storage. This revolutionized the icebox industry and made it more affordable, and more importantly, more accessible for everyone, especially those in the southern regions where freezing outdoor temperatures are rare. Now everyone could have an affordable icebox.

Eventually, appliance manufacturers found ways to greatly reduce the size of the refrigeration compressor units to a small enough size that they were somewhat portable, thus allowing electrical refrigeration in the form of a "fridge" in every home.

This revolution in refrigeration greatly changed the world and how we store and make food. In days of old, some may remember that the size of an electric fridge was considerably smaller than they are today. People didn't have near the amount of food stored the way we do today. Many people also had "root cellars" where they stored the harvest from *their garden*, food on which they would mostly live until the next year's harvest. And when they did have a root cellar and had a good year with an abundant harvest, we have to realize that they had to do a great deal of work for that to occur, so their calorie usage balanced better with what they ate. In fact, for many people in the days of old, they had a difficult time keeping the weight on and many would try to fatten up a bit before winter set in, but they had a tough time doing that because they were burning so many calories as they would prepare for those coming winter months.

Fast forward to today, and we have more food in most of our refrigerators on any one day than most families would have used in a month back then. We live in a time of excess and vast luxury today. Even the poorest-of-poor in America today have at least one TV and a refrigerator and a smartphone with internet. As we all live in the lap of luxury, we have to realize that our world, our culture, and our habits are constantly changing in relation to each other. And if we are not vigilant in taking note and saying "no, thank you" when offered forty-ounce chilled iceless sodas, then we have no one to blame but ourselves.

Just as we abuse the foods we eat, so too we abuse our modern technology, filling our refrigerators with all the wrong things.

Changes in Food over the Years

Refrigeration is one of the most useful and wonderful inventions in the past few hundred years. Refrigeration has revolutionized the food industry, making everyone safer and foods last much longer *without* dangerous decomposition bacteria starting earlier than expected. Many people suffered from food poisoning without really realizing it years ago, but that has mostly vanished with modern refrigeration that allows us to keep our food cool and safe.

Food processing methods have also changed to the point where foods can be freeze-dried and shelved for very long periods in our modern times. In addition to refrigeration, many other manufacturing methods requiring refrigeration have been developed that allow us to have an abundant selection of food in every store in every city, offering us what appears to be unlimited selection and quantity. Today, anyone can walk into any store and buy enough food for a year and store it in their freezer and fridge and pantry and have it last the whole year with very few extra trips to the market if they so choose. We all realize that is not how we do it, but the fact remains that we could store that much that long in our modern world.

But what is worse is that we store great amounts of food in our homes *plus* we go to the market every week or two in addition to that. The problem with this is that it brings the market into our kitchen, which is a good thing if you have super-strength will-power, but if you are like the rest of us, then it can be a real problem. What we choose to buy from the store and keep in our homes is a problem that runs neck-and-neck with our portions sizes that are too large that we choose when we eat from the fast-food drive-thru. And this is only the beginning of these abundant food problems.

Refrigeration is one thing that has allowed us to stockpile unnecessary food in our homes, then add to that that we have vast supermarkets and fast food choices, plus convenience foods *nearly everywhere* a purchase can be made.

And we can go a bit deeper and look at how our foods are made. Most, and even all, foods are great and have some health benefits, yes, even the "junk" foods. But what was meant as a *treat* has become a *food staple* for far too many of us.

The manufacturers obviously make foods as delicious as possible so that we will buy them again the next time we visit the store. Is this some evil plot to destroy us all? No, it is a logical business activity that nearly every one of us would do if we were in that same position and wanted to actually turn a profit so that we could stay in business for the long-haul. There are far too many of us complaining about companies putting this or that in our food so that it is more agreeable to us. So to those complainers I ask, what would you have the companies do? Put soap in everything so that it becomes so undesirable to point that no one buys it?

Let's be realistic. Nearly everything that is put in our foods is there to make our lives better and more enjoyable and safer. Our problem is that we enjoy it all a bit too much, and that's really all there is to it. Since the advent of abundant corn syrup use in our foods as sweeteners, it seems that we have all been gaining so much weight, so some people then try to blame corn syrup use for our fat gain issues. Does that affect our waistlines? Yes, it certainly does, as would using sugar or drinking the equivalent in fresh squeezed orange, apple, or grape juice. Blame, blame, blame. It's always everyone else's fault—When it's really our own fault.

Sure, foods changed over the years and they have generally gotten safer, better tasting, longer lasting on the shelf, less expensive relative to our income, and readily available everywhere. As election time nears, we hear a lot of politicians bemoan the evil businesses and how greedy they are and how people are being starved in their poverty; but this is rarely true in our modern times. People who are suffering from poverty are no longer too thin and malnourished from starvation; in fact it is quite the opposite. Now people of poverty often gain too much weight due to the low prices and abundance of food in the stores, along with free or very low-cost foods from the charity pantries. Unfortunately for poverty-stricken people, the highest calorie foods tend to be the least expensive and so those are the foods that tend to be consumed at higher rates in low-income areas.

Some foods are higher in calories than they need to be, but if we would all stop buying those high calorie items that we love to complain about, then the makers of those foods would no longer make them because they wouldn't sell any if we didn't buy such foods.

Foods are simply better, cheaper, longer-lasting, and often heathier than they were years ago, and we all have adopted the bad habit of overindulgence, or better stated, *gluttony*, and we did so of our own free will. No one held us hostage and demanded that we eat, eat, eat! No, we did this on our own, and the only way out is to begin to fully realize how our bodies work and to understand that the market flows as we demand it to flow. Buy big drinks, and they will offer big drinks—and drink them we will! And ***that*** is how we all got so fat.

We have taken all of these wonderful inventions and abused them, and then we blame the manufacturers for our inability to moderate our desires for these wonderful inventions. The sad part about all of this is that we could enjoy all of what we have ***and*** stay healthy and thin as is intended, *by simply having less* when we have any.

Chapter 5

Breath of Silent Techniques

The functions of our amazing body-machines seem to have no end. There are many very small functions that serve great purpose that most of us will never know or even care about, but these bodily functions dictate what our bodies will do with the foods we eat. When we understand some of these basic functions, then it makes ridding ourselves of that annoying excess fat far easier and far faster than trying to do so without that knowledge. Yet, there are many people who already have that knowledge and still can't lose the fat-weight they want to lose. What's the problem then? It is our lack of wisdom–especially our cumulative societal wisdom.

I Just Want to Lose Weight... Now!

Many of us... No most, if not all, of us just want to lose weight ***now***! But we really don't want to lose weight. What we really want is to lose our excess fat. This might surprise many people, but if you think of it like this it will clear things up a bit; I am willing to bet that if your body looked like you imagine it to look, then you really would not care if you weighed three hundred pounds. But we have a difficult time separating these issues, and so we are always stuck focusing on those pesky scale numbers. Yes, the numbers do matter, but the "but" in this is that it is the *fat* that we want gone rather than the *weight*.

When we "diet", the first couple of weeks appear to be a glorious time when the weight comes flying off and we feel like we will be done in a couple months, but as discussed in a previous chapter, little or none of that weight lost the first two weeks is actually fat-weight loss. And because of the way our bodies work, it is very difficult to lose fat until the body's digestive system has been mostly emptied.

Here is how your system works: Food and drinks are energy, and laboratories have done a great deal of work in finding out how much energy each ingredient has. Our bodies obey nature and the laws of physics and thermodynamics, meaning that our bodies will use that energy as they see fit based upon how much we eat, what we eat, how often we eat, and how much activity and exercise we do each day.

As we consume foods, we chew it up and swallow it, and that is then plunked into the acidic brew in the stomach to begin the digestion journey through our amazing intestines. As this food is broken down with the acids, it is then available to be absorbed through the walls of our stomachs and our intestines. The blood that courses through each one of us passes by the inner wall of the stomach and intestines allowing the blood cells capture the broken-down food nutrients which are then carried throughout our bodies. Our bodies will take whatever they need in order to do their best to rebuild all of the parts of our bodies. Then as we breathe, we introduce oxygen into our blood through our lungs. This oxygen is also carried throughout our entire body in conjunction with the foods that we have already consumed, thus allowing us to have enough energy to function. If we do not have enough food molecules coursing through our system, then our system is forced to take the required energy from our stored fat and from our muscle.

If you fail to get proper foods, then your system becomes starved for critical items and must dig through lots of unneeded items to find just a few required nutrients. Our digestive system can slow down somewhat in cases where we lack proper nutrition, even though we are eating a lot of food. The reason for this is that our bodies need and crave the body's required nutrients needed for proper health. If we short our bodies and only give our bodies low nutrient foods, then our intestines tend to hang on to the food a bit longer while trying desperately to find the particular nutrition the body really needs. You could think of this like trying to build a house using only boards and bricks but no mortar or nails. The house will blow down in the first wind, so to build it up more, you will need to add many more bricks and boards to keep it together. Our fat is the result of two things: eating too much *and **not*** eating the right amount of proper nutrients.

Proper fat-loss comes with reasonable eating, both in quantity and *quality*. There is no reason to demonize *any* foods, they are all great. All we need to do is to take in reasonable quantities of them and also to make sure we are getting our required nutrients each day when we eat.

What to Do

DreamThin is not about exercise, but exercise does help a great deal, especially when you have a long road ahead. We often hear "Exercise a particular exercise till you feel that burn. Then push a bit more, but don't hurt yourself. You may feel sore the first week or so till your body gets used to your new workout." This is not bad and exercise will certainly speed up the fat loss process. But how many people do you know who spend much time every day exercising, but they either are not losing fat or worse, they are gaining fat-weight? Too many is my guess. Or consider some construction workers, these people burn several thousand calories per day depending upon their specific duties, and could potentially lose a pound per day burning that many calories, yet many of them are still overweight.

So apparently exercise is not the real solution to our fat problems. Our bodies can absorb a lot more calories than we would like them to, and our bodies can only burn a few hundred calories an hour while running full speed. That amount of exercise for an hour is roughly about two twelve-ounce sodas worth of calories. That means that if you are eating at equilibrium and are maintaining your weight and then you decide to adopt the habit of drinking two twelve-ounce sodas per day, then you will likely gain a pound every month or two. So, if you wanted your two sodas per day and did not want to gain any weight, you would then have to run for about an hour per day in addition to your current day-to-day habits. That's the reality, and there is nothing we can do to change this simple law of nature. "Eating at equilibrium" is when the amount of daily calories consumed is equal to your daily calories burned, thus causing your weight to remain stable.

It doesn't benefit us a whole lot to exercise for an hour for the purpose of fat-weight loss if we are going to sabotage that effort by rewarding ourselves with a two to four hundred calorie treat.

Clearing of the System

The concept of DreamThin is to be able to lose weight while sleeping *and* without being forced to change your daily activity habits. Losing weight with exercise is possible, and additional exercise is very helpful when you have made sure to check with your nutritionist-physician for safe activity levels for you. But the reality is that we all picture ourselves going for it and exercising until we look like we want to look, or like we did twenty or so years back, yet we never actually stick to it— except of course for those determined few who are able to stick with it and be victorious.

But for the rest of us, the reality is that we just don't want to exercise, even though we know we should. Here's the good news, it takes longer to lose the fat without it, but exercise is *not* a requirement to lose weight. Exercise does speed things up for sure, and it is typically good for your health when done right.

If you're serious about fat loss, then the first thing that needs to be done is to clear your system naturally, no fancy tricks, no laxatives, and nothing unusual is required. Just eat less and eat foods that will make your restroom habits "regular". Often, when beginning to lose weight, the intestinal system is typically filled full, and yet we simply do not feel the need to use the restroom. This situation is not good, especially when trying to lose weight. Our bodies are far healthier when we get enough fruits and vegetables, which help the digestive system function normally as designed.

But don't confuse reduced trips to the restroom with constipation as you reduce your eating to proper healthy levels. Too many of us are lured by all of the hype regarding our health and we are told "if you are healthy, you should poo once or twice per day". But if you don't eat much, then this will change and it might be every other day. Less-in-less-out is a good way to think about it. But on the other hand, if we over-eat and we are not going to the restroom daily, then that can be very problematic for our health. When food sits stagnant in our digestive system for too long it becomes toxic to us and we begin to feel lethargic and all around awful. But when our system clears a bit, then we quickly begin to feel better.

Once our calorie intake, or food and drink intake, has been reduced to reasonable levels and we increase our fruits and veggies, then after about two weeks we will begin to notice true fat-weight loss. When we use DreamThin Averaging for recording our weight as mentioned earlier, then after about two to three weeks we will see the real fat-weight loss begin to show up properly on the scale's readout as we proceed with our goal.

DreamThin is about a type of personal awareness that allows you to be in full control of your fat. Control doesn't come easy with us because we choose to hear anything our itching ears want to hear. If someone tells us that we can eat as we do and still lose weight, then we will listen and obey until we find out that it is not true, at which point we seek another "New and Improved" nonsensical program to follow.

Unless you are perfectly honest and very well acquainted with your calorie count, the chances that you are accurately tallying your calorie intake are about zero. Our ability to lie to ourselves runs deep and wide. This is why it is so important to record your calories daily until you get a very accurate and very solid grasp on how many calories are in the various foods and drinks that you prefer to consume. Fat loss is more of a mental adjustment than it is anything else, and until we accept the fact that real fat loss doesn't begin until after we have cleared our system, we are really not losing much actual fat, if any.

Doing It Right

One of the common problems that many of us run into, even when we do things right, is that we might clear our system properly and actually begin to lose weight, but then in our haste to get things moving along we choose to do extreme exercising. This isn't always a bad thing, for instance if you know what you are doing and are properly trained regarding safe exercise levels and methods and you understand fully your own safe exercise limits, then intense proper exercise can be beneficial. But for the rest of us, we generally don't know our limits. Most of us won't ever even try to get anywhere near those limits because we refuse to get much, if any, activity at all. Yet too many of us give it everything we have, as if we are still sixteen years old, but then we end up injuring ourselves and sabotage our fat loss efforts. Don't hurt yourself exercising!!!

If you choose to exercise, take it easy at first, and safely work up to a more vigorous routine and follow your physician's or trainer's suggestions. Just don't hurt yourself while working to lose fat. If you hurt yourself, you sabotage your progress and can no longer get the exercise you want until after your injury heals. There is nothing that will stop the momentum of healthy progress of fat-weight loss like an injury.

When you exercise, do it right and keep accurate track of your workout time and calories burned. It's generally a good idea to underestimate the number of calories you have used during exercise, rather than over-estimating. We all tend to round up rather than rounding our numbers down when we calculate our calories used, but when it comes to the calories we eat then we conveniently tend to round down–Doing so works against you.

Importance of Accuracy

During exercise or eating, accuracy is very important. At first, recording calories a nuisance, but usually within about a two to three-week period we all have eaten most of our favorite and common foods and have entered them all into our personal calorie guide. After you have recorded the typical foods or meals that you have eaten, group those foods into meals and enter those on copies of the Favorite Foods pages in the back of this book as a reference so as not to have to re-lookup each component of a meal, this way the calories for your common meal items are a ready reference for you.

It generally takes about two to three weeks of looking everything up and writing it in the Favorite Foods pages to accumulate the bulk of the items a typical person eats overall. Your less-common items will have to be filled in as you eat them and record them. It's a tedious task the first few weeks, but it is soon worth every DreamThin penny.

How to Stay in Control... Forever

If you have been fatter than you would like to be for more than a decade, then you probably have been through several diets and have already learned some of what we are talking about in this book. Yet with all of what you have already learned you still can't rid yourself of the unwanted fat.

When we come to the understanding that fat is *stored energy* it clears things up quite a bit. *Control* is as much about *understanding* your body and foods, as it is about self-control. We often think of knowledge as the key to success, but most of us know plenty of people who have had higher education, yet have no sense about them. Rather it is our *understanding* of the knowledge we have that is important, and our *understanding* is more important to us than the knowledge itself is. Without us *understanding*, the "knowledge" is useless, and it is sometimes dangerous trivia to us in that case. In our high-tech culture anyone can find nearly any information online in mere moments, but without understanding, most of it is of little use to us.

We can know the idea that fat is stored energy, but to understand and to grasp that in an internal mental way gives you power over it. As we age, most of us will recall times in our lives that we suddenly had a personal revelation about some piece of knowledge that we had in our heads for many years. But even though we held this knowledge within us, it was useless to us until the revelation came to us personally regarding the meaning of that knowledge. It is *understanding* that then allows us to use that knowledge to change something big or small in our lives.

Take the Bible as an example. It is full of knowledge and we can read it ten times through, but out of the blue one day a verse will come to mind in a certain way and we then understand what was really meant by that verse. Up until that particular point of awareness about that particular verse, it was just knowledge noise to us, but with our personal revelation about it, we can make a change to better suit our intended life direction.

In order to stay in control forever, we must grasp the meaning of the numbers and the inner workings of the human body's ability to process the energy stored as fat. *Accurately* count your calories until it is a mental habit. Be aware of what you eat and do. And chew your food very well!

Be Constant and Be Patient

For most of us we have gained our fat slowly over a long period of time. Most people born before the foods and fast food revolution generally only gained fat after finishing high school, but for far too many young people in this modern era, excess fat-weight gain began shortly after birth.

In years past, gaining fat was generally a very long slow process that was barely noticed, and when it did happen it was attributed to aging. But gaining fat weight is not an issue of aging, rather, it is an issue of habits. Depending upon what we ate and how much we ate and our level of daily exercise, we gained weight at a different pace than others who also have a fat-weight problem. Some people gain the fat-weight very quickly, but that is usually the exception rather than the rule. Most weight accumulates slowly over years, and because it is slow, we keep readjusting our toleration levels of the weight we have gained. Aside of adjusting for a woman's pregnancy or unusual late age growth spurts, fully-grown adults should generally never need to buy new clothing due to having grown out of them. No, as fully-grown adults, our first sign that action needs to be taken by us personally is that our clothing no longer fits. As fully-grown adults, our clothing that we could once easily buttonm but no longer can, is screaming at us that it is time to lose the fat.

These slow changes regarding our fat-weight work both ways. Just as it took time to gain the fat-weight, *it also takes time to lose* the fat-weight. This is why *understanding* our own body is so very important. There is no need for us study and have the full knowledge doctors have in order for us to lose fat-weight, rather just basic understanding of the way our bodies work is usually all that it takes. When we know and understand this, then we understand that we are not going to approach a fat-weight loss effort by wrongly thinking we will be done in only a couple of months.

If anyone thinks they can safely lose that excess forty pounds in a few weeks, then they are sadly mistaken. Proper fat-weight loss is a slow and constant task that requires your patience when you want long-term lasting success.

Here's some good news: If you put on the weight over a period of ten years, it won't take that long to get rid of it when you do it right. Many people can easily shed a half pound or more of fat per week, and even more if they are determined in their efforts. If you start today and take your time, you can lose a couple of pounds per month and in two years' time you will have that fifty pounds gone with little or no extra work. Be constant and be patient and proper in all of your efforts and then you *will* see success!

We need constancy rather than doing it fast, because if we were to run ten hours per day we could theoretically lose a pound per day, but we would probably injure ourselves before the first day is done. And besides, few people have that much spare time to exercise. We are best to do things slowly and consistently and properly, then eventually, with our new habits, the weight will come off naturally and it will stay off permanently because we made slight changes to our life habits.

Chapter 6

Adding Up the Costs

It's surprising how many of us never add up the costs of life. Many of us experience a point in life where we struggle financially and we eventually come to the realization that when things were financially good, we nickeled-and-dimed our wallets and spent a great deal of cash on meaningless items and convenience. Those little things add up!

If you choose to visit the local coffee-house drive-thru, you probably spend a few bucks for a simple drink. If you do that every day during the work week for a year, you have wasted roughly eight hundred dollars and have probably gained some weight from it because it was likely not just a simple coffee, but rather some sugar-laden latte. The same is true if you have a daily soda on the way to work every day. Stop in at a gas station and pay a few bucks for a drink, plus tax, and now you spent about five hundred dollars in a year and probably gained a couple of pounds along with it.

Our habits are costly and must be tamed if we want a long healthy life. There is no need for anyone to join the irritating food-nazi-brigade, rather, we just need to gain a sense of what we are all doing to ourselves and realize just how much our actions and habits are costing us. Be keenly aware of this and use your awareness to stop yourself from doing it every single day of the work-week. Just reducing that alone could potentially reduce many people's fat-weight. But the calories consumed and money spent for that unneeded daily latte, are not your biggest cost.

Medical Healthcare Costs of Being Fat

We also have to consider the medical healthcare costs of being fat. When we are over fat-weight our bodies are being physically taxed/stressed, and due to that stress, we end up taking lots of medication. Some of this medication is simple, for instance, antacids. But for severe cases of indigestion they now make prescription medication to try to remedy a problem that will typically vanish simply by us correcting our eating and drinking habits.

There are many complications that are closely associated with being over fat-weight. The endless doctor's visits and medications and tests add up to a whole lot of money. Sure, you think you don't pay for this because you have great insurance from work, but you do pay and you pay dearly! If we think for a moment that our employers are beneficent contributors to our health costs, think again! The five to fifteen thousand dollars that we cost our employers in insurance early in the twenty-first century would likely be coming to us directly if we were all not as fat as we are today. But as our culture would have it, we have societally created a medical money-eating monster that we are now unable to tame.

You might have great insurance, but then you complain when you have to pay your five-hundred-dollar deductible. You realize that it costs you because you understand that you are fat and the visits are mostly related to fat-weight issues. But regarding costs, consider this common example: wages often stagnate and many politicians then scream about wage stagnation and how wages have not gone up much in the past few decades. This attention-grabbing alarmism is an outright lie. There was a time, not so long ago, that few, if any, people received any insurance benefits from their employers and generally did not need it. But now insurance is a common benefit and thought to be a "right" that must be given to us. Don't get me started on that topic. The cost of insurance per employee is staggering and, in many cases, would increase people's wages by close to twenty percent if the insurance premiums went directly to the people.

The medical costs for our societal fat problem are hidden from us because we are insured by our employers and never really have to deal with the real actual money from our medical bills. The collective national medical expense is pooled into insurance groups and into government "entitlements". This money is then taken from us in a somewhat hidden manner, and is then paid to the hospitals and doctors on our behalf. Because we pay this without really realizing it, we personally never take note that we have a serious health problem. And the part about this that is very unfair to those who are physically fit and disciplined enough to stay healthy, is that they incur little or no medical costs but have to pay near the same cost for insurance and taxes as those of us who cause the problem. If everyone was as fat as the rest of us and visited the doctor for fat-related issues, then our insurance rates would explode to numbers we would rather not think about.

Our wages have increased, but us ignoring the cost to our employers regarding our insurance, is foolish, blind, and ignorant. Pay attention to the insurance value that is taken, yes *taken*, from *your* pay, and realize that those high numbers are largely due to our societal fat problem.

Health Costs of Being Fat

Besides the financial medical healthcare costs of being fat, we also must consider the physical health costs of being fat. Quality of life is often confused with *just being alive,* which is often outright lost in the confusion. There are many of us that don't have a clear distinction that there is a difference between *being alive* and our *quality of life.* Instead we go to a doctor with hopes of having the doctor be able to remedy our self-inflicted problems, and that cost is high, as was mentioned before. But the real cost to us is the discomfort the treatments cause us.

When we have a simple problem like near constant indigestion, then we typically try using antacids, which might work for a while, but then as our habits increase in intensity and we gain weight, we go to the doctor because the antacids are no longer as effective as they once were, so the doctor gives us a prescription for something that is supposed to be more effective for our self-induced indigestion problems. Sure, the prescriptions are expensive, but here we are considering that the reason we are spending the money for the prescription is that we are very uncomfortable, in fact we are so uncomfortable that we made an expensive appointment to see an expensive doctor who will prescribe expensive medication for us. Our indigestion discomfort is so bad that we are willing to spend all of that money just to relieve our discomfort. *That* is a *quality-of-life* issue.

We are willing to pay all of that money just to feel comfortable again. We tend to go into the doctor with the thought of being healed, but much of modern medicine is *not* designed to *heal* us, it is designed to *reduce our discomfort.* ***True healing*** will stop the problem to a point that any medication is no longer needed. What we want in our lives is to be healed, and you can pretty much be guaranteed that in this case, we can heal ourselves if we would only believe enough to cause us to take the appropriate actions regarding our eating habits for that to occur.

The issue of indigestion is very common when we have bad eating habits, and it doesn't really matter whether we are fat or even if we are reasonably thin, but that's only the tip of the iceberg. There are many inconveniences that being overweight cause besides the many other health issues that make us very uncomfortable, these added inconveniences are due to the size of our waist.

We have to consider that when we get too far over fat-weight, simple things like getting into the car can be a challenge for some of us, and often items such as seatbelt extenders are even needed.

Strictly Financial Aspects of Being Fat

Medical expenses of being over-fat typically run high, but the incidental costs are equally as bad or worse. Being fat is not good business for us as individuals. But it pads the pockets of manufacturers, doctors, and hospitals, but that's not their fault, it's ours.

How expensive is being fat? Consider what jobs we are incapable of as our size increases. When we have too much excess weight we have a more difficult time going up and down stairs and carrying things. These sorts of petty issues add up and cause us to be less capable of doing things we would like to do, so we no longer even entertain the thoughts of doing them. Then we have to consider that when we walk into a job interview that we are being scanned by the interviewer to see if we are a good fit for the company. Most companies are going to do their best to avoid us the fatter we get. And only when the employer is having a truly difficult time finding qualified people, will they consider the heavier qualified people.

Is it unfair that an employer would discriminate against us because we are too heavy? No, it's just wise business. If you were an employer who had to choose between two potential employees of equal skill and intellect, one who is healthy and fit and the other who is overweight and struggles a bit to move around, you would most likely accept the fit person because of the lower costs to your business. If a business offers insurance, then hiring a qualified over fat-weight person can potentially drive up the insurance costs of the company. Additionally, certain accommodations might need to be made for the larger employee. So it is just good business to have a healthy staff. And that is just the job aspect of the cost, but we also have to consider that our food costs increase, and our medical costs increase, and our clothing costs increase etc. We can be as smart as anyone, but when our fat-weight gets out of hand, it affects our lives and costs us dearly!

Become Aware

Most of us don't stop to wonder "why?": "Why does my back hurt?", or "Why do I have high blood pressure?", or "Why can't I get hired?", or "Why can't I find a boyfriend?", or "Why can't I find a girlfriend?" Those and so many other costs are the cost of our problems regarding being over fat-weight. It is our awareness of the seemingly unconnected costs that helps us to quickly change our behavior.

Let's take our posture as an example. Sitting in a position with your foot under your other leg's thigh might not be a problem for someone who is at a healthy thin weight, but when we are over fat-weight then the excess fat behind the knee can slightly push the knee apart causing some pain afterwards. This sort of knee pain can then be misunderstood by doctors, because if we don't realize that this can occur due to posture, then we never think to mention it to them. But in this case, a simple change of habits will make the knee pain vanish in just a few days. If we were not over fat-weight then it would likely not have occurred to begin with. Sitting on your foot is just one small example, but posture habits for over fat-weight people cause a great deal of pain and suffering, leading to tremendous medical expenses and unnecessary risky procedures and expensive prescription medications.

There was a time that a family doctor knew you well and would tell you if you were getting too fat. But with our automated modern medical infrastructure, we are, for the most part, all just numbers in a system of statistics. Most doctors do the job with precision, but the problem is that they don't know us today like doctors did decades ago. Nowadays, we go to one specialist for this and another specialist for that, creating a disconnect in our personal medical care. This makes it even easier for something as simple as a posture issue to be a bit more difficult to detect. And thus, we are prescribed dangerous medications for an ailment that is caused by a little too much fat in the area behind our knee when we sit on our foot, something we might have been doing all of our life while reading or watching TV.

There are many insignificant little things like sitting on your foot that people experience but never connect the dots from the ailment to the causing action, and these sorts of issues are more common in those of us who are over fat-weight. Being over fat-weight changes some of the range of movements of our bodies, and it is our awareness of these little things that not only saves us from unwanted pain, but it can also make us aware that we need to take immediate action and do something about our fat-weight.

Just as our clothing getting too tight as we gain fat is a sign that it's time to take healthy action regarding losing fat, so too are the unexplained ailments that send us to perplexed doctors who have, all too often, been trained to throw prescription medication at our health problems.

Most "aging" ailments are more from being overweight than they are from aging. We tend not to notice the fat-weight gain because it usually comes on slow over a long period, maybe twenty or thirty years or more. But as we gain our excess fat-weigh, that fat slowly starts to strain our system and entire our body. Be aware that too much body-fat holds and assists cancer causing toxins, it stresses our joints, and it has many more very negative effects on our bodies.

Get that Control Back

It is time for all of us to take the control of our bodies back from our foolish selves. As we allowed ourselves to gain fat-weight, we lost control of our health and opened the door to many new and unwanted health problems that the pharmaceutical companies are all too happy to try to help us hide by selling us their costly prescription medications. Most of us don't realize how many illnesses and diseases are fat-weight related problems that are instead being attributed to changes due to us aging. This is because we typically get fatter as we get older, thus giving us the wrong impression. Some businesses depend on this, and they are in no rush to spread the word of truth because it's not really good for their business model or their cash flow.

No doctor, no nurse, no hospital, or any other business or person making money from our excess fat has any *financial* incentive to have us change our habits. We have become so big that they consider us their cash cows. We have become a herd of cash cows that have expanded the medical industry to vast proportions never imagined decades ago. We must each take our control back and we must to do it with care and determination. *We are as we eat.* Eat little and be little, eat a large and be large–that choice is yours and yours alone!

There is a fight within us against ourselves to overcome this one single weakness. We *can* control ourselves evermore and conquer our *self.* When we accomplish this, we will find that we also become better in many other aspects of life, because when we take control of ourselves, we then begin to see the richness within the world and realize what can be. Then we can succeed in almost every good thing we attempt.

When we DreamThin we can go from where we are, to where we want to be with accuracy when we are honest with ourselves and our recording of food calories, along with following basic healthy eating practices.

DreamThin Truth gives us the power to make our own decisions, allowing for efficient removal of our excess body fat. When our body fat-weight is gone, then continuing to record our foods the DreamThin way serves as a guide to help steady our habits with direction and order so that we can regain and maintain the balance we once had until it becomes our normal habit again. After that balance is understood and has been achieved, then we are ready to do it on our own and we will no longer require recording our daily habits. Yet, many people do find it helpful to continue recording for the long-term because it helps them keep all of this in mind so that they don't backslide.

Though at times it seems impossible to rid ourselves of our excess fat-weight, it is not impossible. Every one of us can lose our excess fat-weight by dreaming thin. Every one of us can achieve our personal perfect weight if we seek and then see and accept these truths. Dreaming thin makes it enjoyable and easy to lose our unwanted fat-weight *when we understand* that it is not the *weight* we want to lose, but rather it is the excess *fat-weight* on our body that we want to lose.

Our excess body fat is solar energy stored in food that we have eaten and have stored up in the form of body fat during our life, and the only way to get rid of it is to DreamThin, because that is just the way our bodies work. When we believe that we can do this and we DreamThin daily, then we can know, with relative precision, what our weight should be and about when we will realistically be able to achieve that weight. And as an added bonus, exercise will speed up the rate of fat-loss allowing us to finish ahead of schedule when we choose to exercise in addition to simple modification of our eating habits.

One area that tends to make us feel as if we have destroyed our progress is our "special occasions". The holidays come creeping up on us and we still have a way to go to hit our fat loss goals, but then we over-eat during the holidays and step on the scale the next day or the next week causing us to feel like giving up again because our weight is much higher than before those holiday occasions. We feel as if we have lost control again, but we really have not.

This is where the importance of DreamThin Averaging comes into play. When we average our daily weights, it smooths out these phantom weight spikes on the scale's readout. Just because we have temporarily overfilled our system with food and retained water, does not mean that we have gained much, if any, actual fat-weight. In fact, often these occasions will prompt our bodies to lose more weight on the scale several days afterwards to below where we were before the special occasions occurred. However, if we do this on a regular basis and give up and continue eating on the days following the special occasions, then we again will gain fat-weight, which is how we got fat in the first place. Let us all become vigilant and look ahead because we all know when most of these occasions are coming up and we can simply compensate the days prior to, or even after, such occasions by eating a bit less and by taking a longer walk or doing more exercise before and/or after the occasions.

Dream Dollars

Various companies have their systems to track calorie consumption. Some try to keep the numbers smaller by giving meals a numeric value, but those meals are expensive and of a specific size, and when following the program properly they work well. But for those of us who want food diversity and want to continue to eat our own favorite foods, that is typically not the most appealing option.

When dreaming yourself thin, the best method is to think of food-energy and fat as if it is money. Swap calories for pennies and then it becomes very relatable as to what exactly is occurring in our bodies. For instance, when tracking our daily calories, we would enter a typical piece of bread as ninety cents ($0.90) if it's ninety calories per slice. A one-hundred thirty calorie soda would be entered as one dollar and thirty cents ($1.30). Every calorie listed on the nutrients label is to be valued at one penny. A typical small cheeseburger is about three dollars and seventy-five cents ($3.75) in DreamThin Dollars.

Part 1–Calculating DreamThin Dollars

Our foods are like our bills, and they pile up in the form of excess body fat. There is no genetic predisposition to being fat, but there is a habitual family predisposition to our eating habits (see *Strong Family - A Foundation of Rock - The Family Repair Manual*). If we have been taught to overspend while growing up, then we will likely experience financial troubles as adults, and eating is no different. As I discuss in detail in the book *Hot Water - Your Perceived Identity - The Life Repair Manual,* we are familiar with what we grow up with, so when we are served certain foods in certain quantities while growing up, then that becomes "normal" to us, and our habit is formed and becomes a normal part of our everyday life.

When we bite off more than we should chew, then we owe more in calories or DreamThin Dollars. Eating more than we should works just like unwanted credit card debt does; if we over spend, then we owe a debt to Fat & Co. to wear around our waist. And every 3500 calories that we overeat is thirty-five dollars that we owe Fat & Co. Those 3500 calories or $35.00 of debt to Fat & Co. are equal to *one full pound* in fat bills around ***your*** waist.

If we overspend by three hundred and fifty dollars, then we will have bought *ten pounds* of fat from Fat & Co. The only way for us to repay Fat & Co. is to spend less and begin *saving* DreamThin Dollars, or we can earn more DreamThin Dollars by working more or exercising a lot, similar to needing to get a second job.

If an average-height man of about 5 feet 10 inches tall weighs two-hundred pounds then he is roughly 42 pounds over-fat-weight. The amount he owes to Fat & Co. is roughly fifteen hundred DreamThin Dollars. 42 pounds x 3500 calories per pound equals 147000 calories or $1470.00. And if an average-height fully grown woman 5 feet 4 inches tall weighs one-hundred-sixty pounds then she is roughly 43 pounds over-fat-weight and her debt to Fat & Co. is just over fifteen hundred DreamThin Dollars. 43 pounds x 3500 calories per pound equals 150500 calories or $1505.00.

Tracking your calories as if the calories are dollars and cents is easy and it is familiar–and it works!

The Goal for each one of us is to be able to reasonably accurately estimate our goal weight. We must have reasonable goals and understand that different body shapes will affect our proper and healthy Dream Weight. Our Dream Weight is best calculated when visiting a nutritionist-physician and, here, it is recommended that you do so.

We often hear conflicting information about the numbers on the scale, where some people will say that the scale doesn't matter at all, but others will say that the numbers on the scale are very important. This apparent chasm between the two points of view depends upon what aspects of our weight and bodies we are discussing, as well as our own psychological perspective.

Because our muscle-build and body structure can vary greatly from person to person, an exact weight number cannot be stated generically-specific and can only be *roughly* estimated. Adult females can typically have a much greater diversity in a healthy weight variation than do men because of the female figure measurements. An average woman about five feet four inches tall will weigh roughly one-hundred to one-hundred-twenty pounds. But if her chest is larger she could be several pounds heavier at her perfect healthy weight than another woman is. Also, some women are built with much smaller waists at their perfect healthy weight and they might also have slightly wider than average hips. Most of these figure types somewhat average out the weight on any one woman, but must be considered when trying to accurately assess the perfect healthy weight of any one individual. These little shape variations in people can add up to a noticeable perfect weight difference from one individual to another.

Additionally, our muscle mass must be considered because very active athletic people, both men and women, will be heavier if they have lot of extra muscle mass. Not because muscle is heavier as some people wrongly believe, that is false information. But rather, it is because muscle has "tone" and stays where it belongs. Fat, on the other hand, just sits there sagging and weighing down our skin.

The way we look when we are at a specific weight can vary greatly depending upon the amount of muscle we have built up and how toned that muscle is. This is not in reference to body-building in any way, but rather is in regard to when we have little muscle and little muscle tone then we can be at a "healthy weight" but still might not have the appearance we desire, which is because we have no muscle tone. When we properly exercise to accomplish our goals, we can weigh the same or even much more than our theoretical "healthy weight" and look and be very physically fit.

To begin a routine to DreamThin we must first do our best to determine a realistic and healthy weight. By "realistic" I mean that the selected weight number is not determined by our laziness or by our unrealistic desires to hit a certain number. Think of this in terms of a woman not wanting to be considered to have "large feet" so she foolishly crams her delicate feet into shoes a size or two too small, ultimately disfiguring her feet as she ages—Yes, it happened, a lot!

On the other end of the weight-loss spectrum, all too often we do things such as knowing that our weight should be, let's say one hundred twenty pounds for a particular woman, but because we don't believe we can ever hit that, we settle for one hundred fifty pounds as our target weight. With this sort of approach, we have pretty much have guaranteed our fat-weight loss failure, ensuring that we will be indebted to Fat & Co. for life.

There are certain truths in life that we must accept and it is those truths that we see and seek but often fail at accomplishing. Though we see and seek them, we personally do not internally believe that we ourselves are capable of achieving what we seek, so we settle, and that settling is essentially our failure.

If someone is far overweight but their proper weight is one-hundred-twenty pounds, as their weight goes down they will eventually pass the one-hundred-fifty-pound mark on the way down. But all too often we stop at the wrong place. Slow and steady to the *proper place* is the safest and most reliable way to dream yourself thin.

We all need to find the approximate healthy weight for our height and gender, and in doing so, we must with total honesty and accuracy consider chest size, figure type, and muscle build, thus allowing us to have a realistic starting point and realistic goals. Once we have achieved that, we can then calculate the debt we have accrued with Fat & Co. and begin to pay that debt off.

How do we pay off the debt? Savings and extra work, just like with everything else in life. Every person is allowed a certain number of daily calories based upon their height, gender, and muscle mass, and if we exceed that number we will slowly get fatter, this is not a question, it is a simple fact and it is fundamental physics and chemistry. This is not some sort of option that we can take a pill or something to remedy. It is a fact of physics and energy that when we consume more than we need for our daily energy needs, then *we will gain fat*. That is why it is so important to understand what our own personal perfect healthy weight should be. With DreamThin we call it personal perfect weight, not as some random imagined number, but rather as an accurate *assessment* of where you personally should be regarding your best and most healthy weight. Without a realistic number, we tend to choose inaccurate figures that can potentially cause us to continue gaining weight until we hit fat-weight equilibrium, if we ever do.

Fat-weight *equilibrium* is when your weight stays stable based upon your weight and energy needs for your particular activity levels when balanced against your eating habits and food consumption. When you are at *equilibrium,* you will neither gain nor lose weight in the long term. If we eat a little too much each day we will gain weight until our weight is such that it requires more energy to move us around, and then when that energy need comes into balance with the energy we consume through eating and drinking, the weight gain will stop again. The weight will not reverse until the energy consumption of food is cut back or the activity levels are increased *without* the food level being increased.

When at rest, an adult body will use roughly somewhere between thirty and eighty calories per hour depending upon height, gender, and muscle amount. Then our additional physical daily activities, such as walking from room to room and climbing stairs etc. will increase those daily energy needs. The national nutritional label figures show a two thousand calorie diet for the average person, but this is greatly in error considering our sedentary activity levels of our modern era. Nor does it account for our frame size and height and gender. So, it is important to understand that the point of reference on the nutritional labels is only that—*a reference point.* We must adjust those daily nutrition numbers for our own actual height and gender.

As a rule of thumb in nearly all cases, a man and woman of the same exact height will typically have a considerable weight differential. A *typical* woman has natural muscle mass smaller than a *typical* man of the same height. Additionally, women will have smaller dimensions of circumference on most parts of the body causing women to weigh considerably less than men.

The first step to DreamThin is to estimate your personal perfect weight and calculate the DreamThin Dollar value of your excess weight by subtracting your perfect weight from your current weight and then multiply that number by 3500. The approximate calorie count for a pound of body fat is roughly 3500 calories.

Remember, each calorie is worth a penny of debt, that is $0.01 owed to Fat & Co. So, if you are 65 pounds over fat-weight then you owe Fat & Co. $2275.00.

A man who weighs 235 pounds, minus his personal perfect weight of 170 pounds, leaves 65 over fat-weight pounds. Being 65 pounds over fat-weight times 3500 calories equals 227,500 calories or 2,275 dollars.

Until the $2275.00 is accurately and completely paid it is technically impossible for you to achieve your personal perfect weight.

235	Current weight
-170	Perfect weight
=65	Pounds over fat-weight

65	Pounds over fat-weight
x 3500	Calories per pound of body fat
=227500	Calories or cents

Or **$2,275.00** in debt to Fat & Co.

Part 2–Be Accurate

An adult male body of a given height or an adult female body of a given height will both require given amounts of energy to function daily and maintain a personal perfect weight. There are many resources to calculate this, but we must be careful to make accurate and realistic estimates of our personal perfect weight. The only thing any index can do is to give a *rough range* to at least get you close to understanding where your personal perfect weight might belong.

Too often we want absolutes with this sort of thing, but every person is different and unless you see a nutrition-specialist who understands proper-health weight you will have to make these estimates on your own.

Following is a target-weight index shown in pounds with an at-rest calorie index to consider, but both are only shown as *rough guidelines* to help find an estimated target-weight for a given height and anatomical gender. You *must* check with your nutritionist-physician or professional trainer to find your own actual accurate weight goal and 24-hour-at-rest calorie usage.

	Female		**Male**	
Height	Target weight	24-hour at-rest calories	Target weight	24-hour at-rest calories
4 feet 6 inches	94	620	111	854
4 feet 7 inches	96	635	114	875
4 feet 8 inches	98	650	117	896
4 feet 9 inches	101	667	119	917
4 feet 10 inches	103	681	122	938
4 feet 11 inches	105	697	125	960
5 feet 0 inches	108	713	128	982
5 feet 1 inch	110	729	131	1004
5 feet 2 inches	113	745	134	1026
5 feet 3 inches	115	761	137	1048
5 feet 4 inches	117	777	140	1070
5 feet 5 inches	120	794	143	1093
5 feet 6 inches	122	810	145	1116
5 feet 7 inches	125	827	148	1139
5 feet 8 inches	128	844	151	1162
5 feet 9 inches	130	861	155	1186
5 feet 10 inches	133	878	158	1209
5 feet 11 inches	135	895	161	1233
6 feet 0 inches	138	913	164	1257
6 feet 1 inch	141	930	167	1281
6 feet 2 inches	143	948	170	1305
6 feet 3 inches	146	966	173	1330
6 feet 4 inches	149	983	177	1354
6 feet 5 inches	151	1002	181	1379
6 feet 6 inches	154	1020	184	1404

Find your *approximate* target weight. Estimating your target weight too high will likely cause you to fail and gain weight, and estimating too low will be dangerous to your health if you ever were to achieve an unhealthy low weight.

There are far too many resources out in the market that have little or no authority in claims made or that have wording that is confusing to the reader. In some cases, readers get incorrect understanding from these sources. "Social Media" can be the worst resource for getting information because there is too much extremism from people who have not understood the science while at the same time presenting themselves as "experts". This is not to say that it is not possible for them to be accurate, but a seventeen-year-old female giving health advice is not necessarily the best of option for "health and exercise" information. Not that the person is wrong when they are that age, but most people are in very good physical condition at the age of seventeen. However, they are not in such good condition because of perseverance, it is because they are still in their early prime of life.

A ninety-year-old that is still in great shape might be a better option to consider when choosing to seek advice on social media. The point here is that there is much inaccurate information available that we should not be listening to, but too many people do this just because the "expert" is young and beautiful, which is what we want to look like.

Start thinking long-term. There is one guarantee I will make to you and it is that we are all aging. So, looking to older people who are in great shape for some guidance has greater potential of offering more health wisdom for you to consider than does getting health information from "experts" who are still in their youth. Even people who are health and fitness gurus die at very young ages, so we must be careful who we listen to regarding health advice. In fact, even this book should not be considered as any sort of advice to do anything and is only here to offer points that you may not have heard before, rather it is here for your consideration only.

Now that you know how to go about calculating your personal perfect weight, subtract it from your current weight and multiply by 3500 pennies or $35.00. This is your debt to Fat & Co. and your goal is to pay it off as soon as is healthily possible.

When recording your current Fat & Co. balance, you must accurately enter the DreamThin Dollars into your account, similar to how you would do it in a typical checkbook, except here you are paying down your debt to Fat & Co. and must do your best to quickly bring your balance to zero.

If your perfect personal weight and size uses 1700 calories every day, then you will deduct $17.00 from your Fat & Co. bill. Then if your daily food consumption was 1500 calories for the day, you then add the $15.00 that you now owe on your Fat & Co. bill. For that day you will have paid off $2.00 of your Fat & Co. bill. To reduce your debt with Fat & Co. you must spend less than you save almost every single day. To speed things up, you can work extra and make other small payments during the day. For instance, a casual 30-minute jog might be another payment of around $1.00 to Fat & Co. But if we stop on the jog to get a "healthy" bagel or muffin, then we will owe Fat & Co. another $2.00, making that jog a $1.00 debt rather than a $1.00 payment.

100	Jog payment calories
-200	Bagel cost
= -100	Calories owed
or $1.00	Owed to Fat & Co.

When calculating your calories, you must be accurate–pennies add up! If you have ever been overdrawn in your checking account, you likely have quickly realized that a penny error can be very costly when things are tight–Pennies matter!

We all have this nasty tendency to underestimate what we eat and overestimate our exercise, but Fat & Co. uses the latest in debt tracking software and the newest computers that cannot be cheated. Fat & Co. knows exactly what you have eaten, even if *you* do not know. Fat & Co. knows exactly how many steps you have taken, how many breaths you have made, and how many times you have blinked, and they calculate it all with pinpoint precision, never ever missing a single penny-calorie. If you cheat, they penalize you with more and more body fat! Make sure your numbers are accurate for everything you consume and for all activity if you plan to ever get out of the debt-grasp that Fat & Co. has on you.

Part 3-Record it All

A typical stick of sugarless chewing gum has about 5 calories. If you want to be serious about this, then *every* calorie needs to be counted. If we skip these little things we will also skip slightly larger things and eventually it all adds up to not being able to pay off that debt to Fat & Co. So even if you fail to record the 5-cent bill for the stick of sugarless gum, Fat & Co. has ***not*** failed to record it. Just like forgetting to make an entry in your checkbook will cause an overdraft, so too will your bill at Fat & Co. increase your waistline. There is no getting around this simple truth of physics, science, and energy–it's just the way we are Created.

Make sure to count every penny because every penny counts. When recording your purchases and payments, you can easily estimate the date that your bill with Fat & Co. will be paid in full. When you reach that point it becomes easy to pay Fat & Co. a little extra now and then so that they owe you on the day ahead of your next birthday or holiday, allowing you to eat whatever you want and as much as you want that day.

Just as over-estimating your exercise payments and under-estimating on your eating bill causes larger than expected debt with Fat & Co., so too will forgetting items or thinking that they don't matter.

Here is one way we all increase that debt: Let's say that you're at equilibrium and have maintained your weight for twenty years, only ever fluctuating a few pounds up or down at any point. Now, regardless of whether or not you are overweight at the point of that equilibrium, at that point if you increase your consumption you ***will*** slowly gain weight.

So here's the problem: You decide to buy a bag of hard candy and you have only a couple pieces per day. A typical caramel flavored sucking candy is about 20 calories. No big deal, right? Maybe. Since you're consuming 2 pieces per day and you had previously been at perfect equilibrium with your current eating and activity habits, these 2 pieces of candy are now adding a paltry 40 cents per workday to your Fat & Co. bill–no problem!

Let's see... about 250 work days in a year times 40 cents is about 100 dollars. Do this for two years and you have increased your debt to Fat & Co. about $200.00. That's over five pounds of fat that Fat & Co. will force you to wear around your waist or on other areas of your body in only two short years. Now do this for a decade and you have a real problem.

Small things matter and if we imagine that sucking *only* two candies and not gaining weight is a reality, think again! This common situation is rare, not because people don't suck on candies all day, rather it is rare because seldom is it *only* a *couple* of 20-calorie candies, typically it's a donut or bagel per day and a latte to go along with it. A donut and a latte is probably in excess of 600 calories or $6.00 owed to Fat & Co. Luckily, for us when we eat far too much there is a point where our bodies simply cannot process all of the excess and it passes through without being fully processed. If this was not the case, then our bagel and latte habit would cause us to gain about a pound per week.

When we're serious about getting into healthy shape, we have to realize that the little things matter–a lot! And Fat & Co. will ***not*** be cheated in any way!

Part 4–Patience

You *understanding* the time that it takes to pay off Fat & Co. is very important. If you have been the same amount overweight for a long time, then you have been at equilibrium the entire time your weight was steady at that amount over fat-weight. If you decide that you want to lose that weight in a given amount of time, then you must first do some realistic calculations. Failing to do so and failing to understand and accept those accurate calculations most frequently results in fat-weight loss failure.

Let's say that we are 60 pounds over fat-weight and we want to lose that weight in only 3 months. That means that we have to lose 20 pounds per month. Is this realistic?

Let's do some more simple calculating. Let's imagine that our at-rest and daily activity uses a total of 1500 calories per day, That is to say that we make a $15 daily payment to Fat & Co. and theoretically eat nothing all day. Since we are 60 pounds overweight, we currently owe Fat & Co $2100.00.

Now, 30 days in a month times $15 dollars daily comes to $450 dollars per month, and 3 months of this totals $1350.00 leaving us with a remaining balance at Fat & Co. of $750.00 that we still need to repay. So, in 3 months' time, we have not eaten a single bite but we are still about 20 pounds over fat-weight. This ***theoretical*** example *does not* include any eating whatsoever *for 3 full months* and *is not safe and should never, ever be done* because doing so would likely kill you. As you can see, it is unrealistic and very unsafe to attempt to lose 60 pounds in three months without any exercise. If you have the money and time and ambition, then a nutritionist/personal trainer can help you to lose the weight reasonably fast, but even then, rapid fat-weight loss can be a serious risk to your health. *Slow*, *constant*, and *easy* is the best method for fat-weight loss. The time to start is always ***now***.

In addition to the inherent dangers with complete starvation diets, doing so actually harms your body by it consuming your muscle. The way the body works is that it amazingly processes any food we consume and does its best to turn that food into bone, blood, muscle, skin, hair, and of course our unwanted fat. But the reverse is true. When we starve ourselves then our body *will take* ***from*** *our body* to sustain life and our bodies will be consumed as needed in order to give nutrition to our vital organs. It's really very amazing when you study the body. Some of this is lightly covered in the book series *The Science of God Volume 4 Day Six - Evolution versus Man - In Our Image.* Patience is so very important to grasp with regard to fat-weight loss. If we starve ourselves, it diminishes our muscle mass and that diminished muscle slows our calorie usage. Our muscles are what burns most of our calories, and if we diminish our muscle mass it then takes even longer to pay off Fat & Co.

Our social media culture has far too many people trying to make being fat an okay way to live, and if that's what you really truly want, then fine, go for it. But don't expect pity from others when you incur medical expenses and cause their insurance to rise because of your laziness to deal with a problem. The world of social media has positioned itself in such a way that when someone properly loses weight and looks great, they are then shamed by all of the lazy people who have nothing better to do than try and stir up trouble and controversy by saying "big is beautiful" and "you're too thin", etc. This foolish championing of being fat is destructive to the physical, emotional, and financial health of the entire nation.

In the modern social media culture, you are damned if you do, and damned if you don't, but in truth you are damaged if you don't lose the weight. So while a ravenous pack of idiots can spout off on social media and shame good people for doing the right thing, the truth still remains that being at a healthy fat-weight puts you in better health and makes you look better, and will most likely extend your lifespan and increase your quality of life.

There are certainly beautiful people who are fat, but they typically are not sought after for their physique. The problem with the big-is-beautiful crowd is that fat people are often unfairly shamed, but typically it is not society doing the shaming. It's usually our own self that is doing the shaming of our own self.

There is no need to feel shame about being over fat-weight, just deal with the problem and pay off Fat & Co. And then realize that being over fat-weight is like having a mortgage that will take time to pay off—The larger the house, then the bigger the mortgage.

Part 5—Relax and Enjoy Life

By saying "Enjoy Life" we are not saying eat, eat, eat, but rather to enjoy life is to stop and realize the gift that life is. You have friends, family, acquaintances, and people in general who enjoy your company if you're not mean to them. Take the time to notice life! Too often when fat-weight is a large part of our life, we get stressed and uptight, only making matters worse. Never get uptight about your weight, just work consistently to properly reduce it, then in time you will hit your desired reasonable personal perfect weight.

Why It is Worth It?

I have never met any person who lost unwanted fat-weight who was displeased with the results of their efforts. The inner joy we feel when we control our fat rather than our fat controlling us is beyond words for most people. When we feel "fat" and can't seem to conquer it, we then tend to feel down or depressed causing us to take refuge in our favorite comfort, which is usually food when fat-weight is the problem. Once you understand how things work and you use DreamThin Averaging and record your daily balance with Fat & Co. you will see progress every few days quite reliably. You understanding how this all comes together can easily remove those depressing moments when the scale mocks your efforts. But when you use DreamThin Averaging you are no longer susceptible to those daily spikes on the scale.

Dreaming yourself thin is worth it because it works, and you can bank on it. When you accurately track your balance, you should be able to calculate how long your *safe path* to losing all of your excess fat will take; and knowing that *realistic* goal will help you to avoid ***un****realistic* goals like in the example given earlier of trying to lose 60 pounds in 3 months. Just because something *could* be done does not mean it *should* be done. What good is fat-weight loss if you're dead or incapacitated from a foolish approach? Consult your nutritionist-physician and do it properly and be safe.

DreamThin is slow, easy, and proper, and it doesn't demand any routine other than simple and *proper* eating–exercise is a bonus!

To DreamThin

What many of us do not know or understand is that it is only when our bodies are shorted the energy they need that our bodies will be able to lose *any* fat. This is a scientific fact, and it is logical. Only when our energy requirements are not being met through limited eating and absorption are our fat stores being withdrawn from.

Just the same as if you are at equilibrium and then begin a habit of sucking on a few candies per day you will *gain* some pounds in a couple of years. So too, if you exercise with a short brisk walk for 10 minutes three times per day will you *lose* some pounds in that same time period ***if*** you *walk for a few minutes instead of* sucking on the candy. However, if two 20-calorie candies are replacing two 200-calorie bagels then things are a bit different, but the math still applies.

One of our biggest fat sins is that we get a latte or a soda and sip on it all day long. This is especially common for those of us with daily desk jobs. We might not even eat all day long just to keep our weight in check, but because we sip that drink all throughout our day we are not able to lose any fat-weight, and instead we tend to gain fat-weight. This is because when we sit at a desk, we are sedentary and we burn very few calories. Then add to that the sipping of the high-calorie drinks all day long, and you will quickly find that it stops our bodies from being able to burn fat calories. If the calorie intake rate from sipping a high calorie drink all day is higher than your at-rest fat-calorie burn rate, then you slowly gain weight just from sipping a seemingly innocent drink throughout the day.

To DreamThin is to have periods during every 24-hour day where your body is forced to burn off fat calories, rather than it directly using food calories during those periods. The premise of "DreamThin" is that most of our weight should come off while we sleep as a natural effect of the body's functions, but because of the foods we eat, the quantity of them that we eat, and also due to ***when*** we eat those foods, we sabotage the body's ability to burn calories while we sleep and dream.

Our world of entertainment is built to sell and tempt us through *advertising*, thus helping the companies that advertise to sell us their products so that they can survive financially and provide jobs for us. Often the entertainment works in conjunction with the advertising, which you will notice when you pay close attention as you see inserted products in those entertainment shows. The point is that they are constantly advertising various foods and drinks as we sit watching, thus prompting us to go into our well-stocked store-like pantry and fridge and select the advertised item, or other similar items, that we were just tempted with in the commercial or in show product placement.

Any evening that we eat several hundred calories just before bedtime causes us to sabotage the body's ability to burn off fat-calories while we sleep. Depending upon what and how much of it you eat, it can take several hours before your body can begin to burn off any fat. When our system is constantly being fed food, it fills our intestines and the intestines will continuously extract the energy from that food and store it as fat. If the intestines are not allowed to be emptied due to our constant eating, then we simply cannot burn the calories of fat that we want to rid ourselves of. Our intestines will extract all of the energy they are able to as long as food is in them.

DreamThin is not about nibbling all day long and eating indiscriminately. DreamThin is about eating reasonably sized meals two or three times per day and causing a slight food calorie deficit, so that Fat & Co. eventually gets paid off. The great part about dreaming thin is that you can make small payments all night long every single night of the week while you sleep when you understand how to do it. There is no additional exercise required, just slow steady progress forward to your personal perfect weight. But you can also Day-DreamThin by understanding how the body works and eating smaller meals so that your fat-burn hours are increased to include some daytime hours as well.

When you have consulted with your nutritionist-physician and you have a good grasp on how DreamThin works, you can increase your rate of fat-weight loss by taking brief brisk walks during those burn times. Doing whatever safe exercise you enjoy for only a few minutes here and there during the day can have a profound positive impact on your fat-weight loss efforts. There is little if any need to workout for hours on end when you understand how your body works and you properly adjust your eating. The reason many of us exercise, and yet cannot lose fat-weight is that we either do not know or we refuse to understand and acknowledge this basic information about losing fat-weight.

To DreamThin you must *understand* your body and the way it works and how food affects it if you want to quickly pay off Fat & Co. the DreamThin way.

Chapter 7

Divide and Multiply Your Biology

Our bodies are incredible machines, and the cells within them are even more incredible. Consider the embryo of a baby: When conception occurs as the single sperm cell penetrates the single egg cell, the most amazing thing begins to occur at the conception moment as a type of spark flashes as discussed in The *Science Of God Volume 4 - Day Six - Evolution versus Man - In Our Image*. Then the cell quickly replicates itself by splitting off and then each cell does the same again and again. This continues all throughout our lives, our cells must divide to multiply and that is how we grow and heal. Without this incredible function we would all cease to be.

What is even more amazing is that once these cells are all in place and continue to multiply, they find a rate of replication that suits us as humans and we then stay roughly the same size and form with the exception of our muscle and fat mass–both of which *we* can control. Then as we eat our foods, these very same cells take the cells and nutrients from the foods we eat and they turn them into muscle, fat, bone, skin, blood, hair, etc. We give little thought to all of this, but it is really most amazing!

Our culture has made the most grievous error in our unspoken understanding of fats and other aspects of the foods that we eat. Sometimes there is maybe too much analysis by "experts" on our human biochemistry regarding what is good or bad for us. It is not so much a matter of what we eat as it is how much we eat *and what we* ***don't*** *eat* that causes our health troubles.

As amazing as our bodies are, they do have certain requirements, but those requirements are often obscured by our freakish unspoken societal misunderstanding of the foods we eat. Manufacturers are going to say and put *anything* on the packaging that is legal that might garner our attention and cause us to purchase their food items. When some "guru of fitness" decries fat in foods as evil, then the manufacturers are going to shout "low-fat this" and "low-fat that". But here is the problem with this low-fat issue: The concerns regarding fat arose because of cholesterol and issues surrounding the heart, but have somehow mysteriously migrated into the dieting and weight loss aspects of life.

It's as if we believe that consuming fat will make us fat and therefore we tend to look for low-fat foods. Fat has little or nothing to do with us getting fat. In fact, in the "Atkins" or keto-type diet, fat is a requirement, where if you do not eat any carbohydrates and only have protein and fat, as much as and as often as you want, then you will actually burn off body fat even though you might be eating vastly more calories than you are burning. And because of the way human biochemistry works, we are incapable of storing fat in that case because we have reached a state of "ketosis". This form of dieting has worked for many people, but it often fails in the long-run because life is pretty boring when you cannot eat carbohydrates.

Consider a cow. Cows are built of muscle, bone, and fat just as we humans are, yet for thousands of years cows were grass fed or fed on corn and corn stalks. Their cow-bodies process those items and turn them into muscle, fat, bone, and hair, etc. The same is true for us. Eating fat does not make us fat, but eating too much of anything typically does make us fat unless we cheat ourselves out of a robust selection of foods and put ourselves into a near constant state of ketosis. There are dangers in any diet, and some diets have more danger than others. But the best diet is the one that gives your body the proper nutrition that it needs overall but is also just short of your daily calorie requirements for equilibrium during the period when you are trying to lose fat-weight. For many people this means that if you are at equilibrium, then nothing more than a couple of brisk 10-minute walks per day will likely cause safe and effective fat-weight loss. It is always recommended to check with a physician when changing your activity levels and/or eating habits.

Food is food. Junk food, fast food, good food, any food, they are all good for us *in **proper** quantities and at proper times.*

Food is Not Evil, Food is a Gift!

Or modern culture, with its excessive opinions on social media, has many of us believing that fast-food joints are evil and that they are *trying* to make us all fat. Well, I am here to tell you that they are not. If we don't like them, then we should shut up and go elsewhere to eat. If we are too undisciplined to handle going to a fast food place and order the health-conscious choices and reasonable portion sizes that they offer, then that's our own problem, it is not everyone else's problem. And it is certainly not the restaurants' fault.

There is really no food that is bad for us, rather it is the ***quantity*** of those foods that are bad. And while manufacturers tend to stick to safe daily limits for a serving size in any one of their food items, our problem is the we don't eat just one single serving, we typically eat several servings. And we also eat at other times of the day and consume near our recommended *daily* amount of calories in a single meal a couple times a day.

There are two perspectives of the nutrient info on the packages. One is that they are saying we need to consume at least this much of each nutrient in a day, and the other is that we should not exceed those daily numbers. Which is true? Both and neither. Both is true because some items like vitamin C can be consumed in very large quantities with little or no adverse effects, while sodium in a similar percent of excess of the recommended maximum dose might briefly cause negative ramifications on our body, even if only temporary. But in truth neither is true, because those numbers are merely guidelines for us in order to give us an *idea* of the amounts of each nutrient we are consuming in any particular product.

We tend to take supplements to compensate for our deficiencies if we are deprived of certain nutrients and this does solve the problem for some people. But the best way to solve nutrient deficiencies is to eat foods that will supply the nutrients that we are deficient in. This is obvious when you think about it in that way.

All foods are a gift! Yes, even junk food *when it is not abused.* A cookie or a candy bar or a piece of cake can bring joy to us if only for a moment, and the health value of that joy far exceeds the calorie addition for that special occasion day. But every day all day is *not* a "special occasion". Our problem is that junk foods were originally introduced as treats, but we have made them our main course. "Junk foods", as we call them, began with the intention of us consuming a serving, maybe two, but we don't consume a serving or two. We consume half the family sized package which is usually about five or six servings. Yes, nearly all of us are guilty of the fat sin of consuming five or six servings all *by ourselves*, and that called is "gluttony".

You need not look far to find someone out in the world who will condemn this food or that food, until all foods are eventually condemned by these various people. One person will swear by fruits and condemn veggies. Another will swear by veggies and condemn meat. Another will swear by meat and condemn fruits. This works for them because they are probably making money from that opinion or have succeeded in losing weight or improving their health with it. But the truth is that it is *all* good food. Those who have improved their health by replacing the condemned food with their chosen food were most likely abusing the particular food they now see as evil, or maybe they had some peculiar allergy to it. *All* foods are good in *proper* quantities!

Fat! Is it a Gift or is it Torture?

Your body has been created with many abilities. It is a literal chemical refinery. If you're an environmentalist, please don't protest yourself, this kind of refinery is very good and very efficient. Our bodies are designed to store energy in the form of body fat for use at a later date. Today is a later date, so let's start using it.

By design, our bodies are doing exactly what we are asking of them to do, which is to consume energy and store the excess energy as fat, or consume less energy and lose fat energy by allowing it to be used to sustain life. The body was made that way for a reason and when you understand that fact and accept it, then you will easily be able to use the energy stored as fat and become the lighter weight you should be and that you desire to be.

The body-fat-storage-system created in you is a sort of reserve system. If you are working out or simply working heavily, your intestines cannot process enough energy quickly enough to supply your muscles' energy requirements, so at that point the fat storage system kicks in and starts to use body fat energy as well as the food energy in your digestive system. This is why when we exercise we must get our heart rate up and sweat a bit to burn fat.

This is the point where our digestive system can't keep up with the energy needs of our bodies and the fat starts to "burn" off.

When we have a lot of food in our system, then shortly after we stop exercising and are at rest, the body's energy needs drop while the energy in our digestive system is still processing. The excess new energy in your digestive system being processed will promptly be put right back where the fat was over the next several hours.

Generally speaking, we are somewhat limited as to the maximum amount of fat we can store in a given day, but there are too many factors to be able to make any sort of accurate estimate. The amount generally ranges between about a half an ounce and about five ounces per day depending upon height, build, what you ate that day, the amount of exercise you did, and the actual overall size in square inches of surface area of your entire digestive tract.

Olympic athletes that train all day long have the luxury of eating as much as they want because their muscles demand more energy than their bodies can absorb from the food they eat. But few if any of us typical members of society want to work out that much. And many athletes will choose nutrient-dense food rather than chips and soda.

Fat is not some torturous thing that some cruel god put on us. Fat is a vitally important aspect of our bodies. A typical healthy adult male will have about 7 to 15 percent body fat, and a typical healthy adult female will have about 10 to 25 percent body fat. In women the extra percent usually has to do with chest, hips, and butt and the fact that the muscle mass is usually somewhat less in women than it is in men of the same height. Fat inside of our torso area protects our organs, and fat on the outside gives us some padding and protection from cold weather.

Fat is what we use when we need some extra energy. Without our fat system we would have to nibble food all day long or we would likely soon die. Fat is a gift, but we have turned it into a plague by accruing too much of it. When our torso area has too much internal fat inside, it tends to choke our organs a bit which causes all sorts of problems, "indigestion" is probably the most common.

What and Why and How that Affects You

If you gain two pounds per year, that is one pound in 182 days, which is about 1/9th of one ounce or about 3 ½ grams per day, or about a half of a teaspoon per day of added Fat. To demonstrate to yourself how little that is, imagine rubbing a half teaspoon of lotion on your hands and you will quickly see that it becomes a pretty thin layer that will not show up on a bathroom scale until you build that layer upon layer for about 15 to 20 days. Even then it might not show up because you may have sweat a lot that day, or you may have just visited the restroom causing your weight to be down a pound or two. Fat comes on slowly until it adds up enough for us to see it on the scale or in the mirror.

A pound of butter is the easiest and most common visualization of how much bigger you are when you gain a pound. But don't let that affect your view of butter. Food items such as butter have been demonized by alarmist researchers who tend to get things wrong and refuse to admit to their errors until the stigma sticks and society succumbs to their lies. And then they will only admit to their error decades later, or they finally die and someone else exposes their lies and/or errors. Butter is one of those items along with eggs that have been defamed and demonized by overzealous researchers and, unfortunately, our government; only later to find out that these things are actually good for your health in reasonable quantities.

I Want to Gain Weight, Not Lose Weight

You might feel that if someone wants to gain weight, but can't, that they are actually very lucky. But I can assure you that if someone is having trouble gaining weight they are probably too thin, and possibly dangerously so and would love to have the ability to gain weight that the rest of us abuse.

If someone needs to gain weight because they are dangerously thin, then either they have some sort of rare medical or mental issue, or more commonly, they have equally bad habits as the rest of us, but in reverse. Some people in this situation think that eating high fat foods is the way, but it is more an issue of eating more than enough of everything on a regular basis.

Personal and family habits are the biggest factors in our personal current condition. It is pretty much a guarantee that if an underweight person eats and moves similar to an overweight person then they will gain weight, barring some peculiar and rare medical condition. Inversely, if an overweight person eats and moves like an underweight person, then they will most certainly lose fat-weight.

But here again we have to consider the meaning of "underweight" and even "overweight". If a guy is a "ninety-pound weakling" he may have the proper percentage of body fat according to all charts, but he has very low muscle mass and the only way for him to increase that muscle mass is to get enough physical activity and eat enough quality foods and slowly build up those muscles. If he doesn't get enough quality calories, then he will be taking from his muscle to sustain life, and in such cases he also has very low body fat, likely too low.

If a newlywed man wants to carry his bride over the threshold he might be incapable if his muscle mass is too low even if she is at a personal perfect weight. When we lack proper nutrition, we suffer the consequences, and that often appears in the form of health problems, one of which is being underweight. When working to gain weight we can eat right and increase our eating and exercise our muscles until we start to gain weight. This might include eating things that you are not accustomed to that have a higher calorie content per bite. But always be cautious to not develop bad eating habits.

Our Bodies Will Seek Needed Nutrients

Our bodies seek certain nutrients and the body is determined to extract those nutrients from whatever we eat. If our food is deficient in important nutrients then our bodies must process unneeded food order to extract enough of what it needs in order to build the various tissue to needed levels. The foods that the body does not need are either stored as fat or are processed and cause unneeded wear and stress on our organs. The body also tends to hold onto our food longer when we are deficient in nutrients in its attempt to extract those nutrients from our current digestive system content, sometimes resulting in constipation.

When our bodies are forced to process more food to extract the required nutrients, they are also processing lots of extra unneeded and unwanted energy, which is plunked down in our bodies in the form of unwanted body fat. Eating fat doesn't make us fat, eating too much of anything makes us fat, but when what we eat is deficient in nutrients, then we suffer many ailments. Our systems need to pass our food through on a reasonably regular basis, and there is really no particular "normal" as to how often we should poo. But when our digestive system is stagnant and nothing is passing through us, it tends to get toxic, only making matters worse when we are nutrient deficient.

Barring some medical condition, we can pretty much eat whatever we want as long as we don't eat too much of it ***and*** we are also getting enough required nutrients to meet the body's daily nutrition needs. We just need to do so in reasonable quantities.

How Much Should I Eat?

How much should I eat? A better question is, how fat do you want to be? We should eat only about as much as our bodies will use in a day. Eat too much and we will gain fat, eat too little and we will lose fat. Over all of the years and through all of the advertised diets, that simple bit of logic has never failed anyone.

When we get enough nutrients and the right number of calories to match our inner build, then over time our weight will come to equilibrium very near to our personal perfect weight. Eat less and lose fat-weight fast, exercise more and lose fat-weight faster yet–Eat healthy and be healthy.

We *can* have our cake and eat it too–if we share it and don't eat the whole thing on our own. And that is the primary point of the DreamThin perspective. We can eat what we like as long as we are getting our required daily nutrients and our calorie count is reasonable and is at or below our personal perfect weight's calories needs. When we put gaps in our eating and eat foods that allow us to have periods where our body is burning our fat at various times during a 24-hour day, especially at night, *then we* ***will*** *lose weight.* The more we short our daily calories, then the more quickly we lose weight. But we must make sure to meet our daily *nutrient* needs.

Count the calories of everything that enters into your body vessel and record them accurately, and then by the time you have accomplished your fat loss goals you will have created a new reasonable level of eating habits for yourself. Plus you will know, at a glance, how many calories most food items are. This allows you to meter what you eat with little or no effort going forward. It becomes second-nature to us and will keep us looking good and healthy as long as we follow the simple science of the body, which is *The Science of God.*

Chapter 8

Things to Know About Your Body

The way we think about our bodies is often affected by our personal beliefs. Some of these beliefs are nothing more than inaccurate perceptions about the way we view ourselves in the mirror. We inaccurately judge ourselves by the way we look. It is true that when we are over fat-weight that there typically are underlying personal issues that we are failing to deal with. But we unfairly allow public perceptions and our own view of our own weight to be our index of our worth as a human being.

Lying to ourselves by saying that "big is beautiful" in order to attempt to boost our personal self-worth is a foolish lie to self, and it only serves to slowly undermine our feelings of worth. Our self-worth should never be tied to our weight, but it is for almost every one of us. When we are over fat-weight we know that we are letting ourselves down, we feel our own self-worth and self-esteem being lowered more and more with every extra bite we take. Big is not beautiful, it is generally unhealthy and no amount of boisterous demanding otherwise on social media is going to change this basic truth, but the person inside of that big body may be a very beautiful person just itching to escape. And "Big is beautiful" is not anyone's pathway to that escape. If someone is comfortable being fat, then that is up to them, but please don't lie to the rest of the world imagining that there is not eventually going to be a financial and health price to pay for being over fat-weight.

We also have the science-world to contend with as they continue ever-devaluing our souls. Our beliefs regarding whether we were Created by a Creator or if we have evolved from monkeys or whatever their latest guess happens to be, has a great deal of impact on our understanding of the way our bodies function and why our bodies do what they do.

When we believe in human evolution, from whatever source they say we came from next, then we devalue our true selves. In the eyes of the Creator we are made in the image of God. What does this mean? It means a lot if you actually study science and the Bible closely.

We are not just some random freak chance beings that randomly formed because some lightning bolt hit some amino acids and then formed us over billions of years. We are Created "in the image of God". This is of great importance in understanding *how*, and more importantly *why*, our bodies work as they do. I get into some basics of this Creation aspect in the book *The Science Of God Volume 4 - Day Six - Evolution versus Man - In Our Image.*

If we are in fact Created, then there is purpose in every element of us. If we have evolved, then *purpose* cannot be considered and we can only try to understand *how* everything works, thus ignoring *why* everything works as it does. *Purpose* is a very important aspect of us and of our fat storage mechanisms.

If nature made us this way, then nature just sucks and we are stuck with it, but if it all has deliberate *purpose*, then we can easily have power over it if we only ask and try. But to do so, we need to learn a couple of basics about our bodily systems. If we are Created, this means that fat has a *purpose* and it is able to be stored for a *purpose*. Knowing that we are Created and that our bodies are "in the image of" and have been designed with purpose gives us an advantage in our fat loss quest. We are designed to work, not to struggle. And many people love and enjoy their work very much. Even though we complain about our jobs sometimes, we generally enjoy the work. The problem is that our bodies are designed to work and move, but many of us don't really do much of the physical *work* that our bodies are designed for. If we were not designed to do things then we'd have a lot less moving parts.

Health of a Nation

Earlier in this book, we discussed a bit about fast-foods and junk foods and then later commented that all food is good, and this is true. But we always have to consider *quantity*. Water is great for our bodies, but if we drink gallons per day it can kill us because it flushes critical nutrients out of our system, thus depriving us of many of the nutrients required to sustain life. So as you can see, something wonderful that we will eventually die without, can also kill us if we abuse consuming it. ***Everything in moderation*** is a really good rule of thumb for all of us to use.

Our problem as a nation is not that all of these wonderful businesses are out there willing to make us burgers for only a couple bucks a per burger; our problem as a nation is that we indulge our desire every chance we get and we will use anything as an excuse to eat again. Fast-food places get an unfair rap from society because it is claimed that their food is "bad" for you. But this is not true, the real problem is that there are so many to choose from that our choice becomes "Which restaurant?" rather than "Should we eat out tonight?"

In years gone by, before the advent of refrigeration, our food chain was short and unstable. All of our amazing advances in food technology have been very good for the health of the nation.

Where before refrigeration and preservatives, our foods suffered and would often go bad, and when food is on edge before it is considered to have gone "bad" it is highly susceptible to insects and parasitic bacteria, thus causing people to get worms as a somewhat common occurrence or even to get food poisoning. There are many such circumstances that have been alleviated by advances in our foods and food storage techniques.

We are often forced to listen to the virtues of eating only organic foods, and I have no problem with doing so, but if you're going to forego an apple because it is not "organic", then you will likely die at an early age because you're so uptight about what you eat that the stress you endure due to this will likely shorten your life considerably.

All food is good! And if we are replacing eating chips, then a non-organic apple is going to be a far better snack choice than no apple at all. The disingenuous advertising in the food delivery chain and all of the experts that demonize every imaginable food are perhaps the most damaging aspect of the health of our nation.

Many people are too busy to study enough to combat all of the bad information out there, and there is also infighting in the food industry for market share of sales. So the juice business might trash the soda business, and soda business might trash the coffee business etc. But the most absurd is when you are made to feel bad for buying a bag of apples that are "**non**-organic".

Let's get serious here, all apples are "organic" and the ones that are well taken care of, be it with pesticide or natural pesticide are better and have less chance of having worms than those that are "organic". The best apples are the ones that are not full of bugs or all beat up. Often "organic" fruits are of poor quality. Clean and well-maintained fruit, whether organic or not organic, is best.

All of this demonizing of foods is relative to what it is being compared against. Some foods are thought of as "super foods" because they are very high in many essential nutrients, and I don't want to take away from that perception, especially when using food for medicinal and curative purposes. But for most of our needs, simply cutting calories and introducing *any* fruits will improve our personal situation—even if that fruit is not "organic".

The Family Disease Lie

To get a bit more into something that was touched on earlier in this book, we are generally *not* predisposed to getting fat or to getting most other diseases because our family has some erred genetic marker showing some predisposition to this disease or that disease. No, our *habits* dictate our health more than anything else does, and that runs nearly equal with our internal beliefs and the stress caused by those beliefs. The beliefs referred to here are not our religious beliefs, though those do affect us, but rather we are referring here to *anything* that we believe and stress over. It has become apparent to me that when someone worries and stresses too much they will often be attacked by that which they stress over. We see this with cancer and heart issues, where someone in the family has a problem and maybe dies because of the disease, but then another family member, usually a child, then becomes so afraid of the disease that the stress on them harms their immune system to a point where the very same disease rapidly attacks them.

The person may indeed have had some sort of family marker in their DNA, but they would never have had a problem if their system was not over-taxed by the very damaging effects of the chemistry that mental and emotional stress causes within our bodies.

Weight gain is one area that scientists claim to see genetic markers, but the *meaning* of the supposed "markers" is really quite another story.

The Genetic Lie

What came first, the chicken or the egg? That is a great question for a book of another topic like the *The Science of God* Volumes. But the premise of the question is the same as the genetic markers issue. What came first, being fat, or the genetic marker for a "predisposition to being fat"?

Science often has a wrong perspective. We see similarities between things and realize that somehow there is some sort of connecting thread, but we then go further and insist that the connecting threads are the *cause of* something rather than *an indicator of*. Nowhere is this more true than in the world of DNA research. An interesting field it is true, but it is highly likely that much of it is misunderstood and is being viewed incorrectly.

Our understanding of facts, figures, and statistics generated in modern science is often frightening, especially when it pertains to our health issues. But let us not place all of the blame on the sciences, because often it is the presentation of information, especially statistics, that clouds any particular topic. Science might create a data set for the world to see, but the groups, businesses, or people with special interests, will take those statistics and present them in a deceptive manner, all while not actually giving false information to us. This is usually done in the realm of *cause* and *effect*, or "the chicken or the egg". What is the *cause*, and what is the *effect*?

The reason that we keep getting fatter as a nation is that we keep believing all of the misinformation and outright lies about our foods and our bodies and the programs that we do in attempt to lose our unwanted fat. When we buy into the erred idea that we have a predisposition to getting fat because of some nonsensical family-obesity fable, then we have bought into a lie that will keep us fat for the rest of our lives.

Most people don't care if someone is fat. We care if *we* are fat, and if we can't lose weight then we tend to take out our frustrations on people who are fit and are in good shape. And in doing so, we say foolish and cruel things to or about them because we are envious or jealous of their success.

We fail to achieve that same success because we choose to believe lies, or at least we believe wrong analysis about things like DNA, thus using it as an excuse to not have to stand strong and do what it takes to lose all of our unwanted fat.

There is no amount of covering our fat sins with "DNA markers" that will reduce our fat. But eating less will reduce our fat no matter what. There is not one single person on this entire planet, and there never was and there never will be, who would not be able to lose body fat when reducing calories to a suitable level–if they really want to and are honest and follow the truths about fat-weight loss. There is just no getting around this simple fact of science and physics. If you track every single calorie that enters your body, and you are honest and accurate about your daily activities and if you reduce your calorie intake below the amount you burn, then *you **will** lose fat.* There is no other option here, it's just how the body works, regardless of the erred interpretation of scientific DNA markers.

The problem that we all have is that we are so lazy regarding disciplining ourselves and our eating and exercise, that we will do anything to make it look as if it's not our own fault. But it is our own fault, and until we stop blaming someone or something else we will remain fat, fatter, and fattest! We are *not* fat because of genetics. Genes are altered by our environment as they now know, and it is highly likely that it is the environment of our over overeating that creates the so-called "fat markers" allegedly found in our DNA.

Family Habits that Cause Our Health Problems

The single biggest reason we keep getting fatter is that we keep believing the agenda-driven scientific-nonsense that allows us to imagine that we are some sort of genetically fat freaks. The world is telling us, "it's not your fault". Wrong! It is our fault, and we're the only ones who can fix it. Just like God wants people to admit they did wrong and for us to stop doing wrong, we must admit to our overeating and stop eating more than needed before we can dream ourselves thin. We need to heal ourselves and forgive ourselves and then move on. The first step is to admit that we eat wrong when we too much.

We are not fat because Mom and/or Dad were fat. And they were not fat because their parents were fat. We are all fat because we eat more than our daily allowance and because we are told the lie that "genetics gave you slow metabolism, therefore you are fat" and we foolishly believe it. How gullible are ***you***?

It is simply a matter of eating a little too much per day for a very long time and gaining only a few grams of body fat each day, an amount that is not readable on any bathroom scale for many weeks. Not even a high-quality industrial grade digital scale can accurately detect a couple of grams of added fat on you per day. Three grams is about a one tenth of an ounce. This means that in ten days you would gain only about one ounce of fat. Most bathroom scales won't notice a three-gram change until there are enough three gram increases to round up to the next digit up. A digital scale with 0.1 accuracy measures in about an ounce and a half or about 43 grams increments. Typical bathroom scales are intended to weigh in pounds and show this decimal amount only for our satisfaction. But those decimal amounts can change just by standing slightly off center on the scale. Our bathroom scales are generally reasonably accurate regarding pounds, but not in relation to ounces.

If we gain only an ounce of fat every ten days, that puts us at about only two ounces of fat gained per month. When we use the restroom, we typically will remove about four times that much waste from our body each time we go. So if we gain three ounces of fat in a month, that would be nine ounces of fat gained in three months. We can fluctuate more than that with a visit to the restroom. That makes it difficult to detect the fat gain even with a very accurate digital scale, which takes us back to the need for DreamThin Averaging.

We also have to consider that while doing something like jogging for an hour, we can easily sweat off over a pound of water weight. So, we gained nine ounces of fat in three months, but we don't fully realize it due to these sorts of fluctuations. If we do this for a year we will have gained roughly two pounds and four ounces.

The reason that this is being rehashed here is that our family *habits* dictate our fatness, our DNA does ***not,*** and too many of us do not want to accept this fact of true science. If you cut the numbers just mentioned in more than half, it is even more difficult to detect the weight gain. You can see in that example just how easy it is for our family habits to cause us to gain weight. If you are a thin growing sixteen-year-old and you are still filling out as you reach adulthood, you can gain a pound of excess fat a year and not notice it because you're still growing. Then, as we age we continue to gain a pound each year. No big deal–until we hit our forties. At that point we realize that we are twenty, thirty, forty or more pounds overweight just because we gained only a pound or so per year.

Family habits that seem insignificant tend sneak up on us and catch us off guard when we are in our thirties and forties. These same family habits that cause us to gain weight are also the culprit for many "family diseases". Anytime we buy into these statistical and analytic inaccuracies, we have submitted ourselves to the mercy of an uncaring medical machine that has lost almost every sense of being the personable service we humans knew and loved throughout most of the twentieth century.

Dangers of Being Overweight

In our contemporary culture, everything is treated as a symptom, and those symptoms are prescribed medication without the doctors having had full knowledge of all of the circumstances in our lives. Much of the prescriptions that are given are over-prescribed, and often additional prescriptions are given to us to counteract the side-effects from the first prescription.

Once we get sucked into this unsafe sewer of medication, we have handed our lives over to a system that has no care or compassion for us and only cares for the money it can extract from the companies and government that insure us. It's not necessarily even the people running it, because it is all just numbers in the system and the only thing that matters to the system is that it gets paid from someone. Then someone, somewhere who knows nothing of the any of the circumstances will demand to be paid, even if the medical establishment made errors in our care and even errors in billing.

Our family habits are *habits* and they are *not* genetic, and those habits are putting many of us in the ground way ahead of schedule. The average lifespan for us is about seventy-seven years, but in truth many people live much longer because seventy-seven years is only an *average* age at death. That means when we die too early we skew those statistics. If the average is seventy-seven then that means that if you die at *fifty*-seven, then, statistically, someone else will live to *ninety*-seven. Here is the sad fact: both people can live healthily until ninety-seven and change the statistics. But because of the many problems associated with being fat, we cause those statistics to be as they are by dying prematurely, and that is the danger of being overweight. But let's call it what it is, over **fat**-weight.

Chapter 9

Health and Mental Protections

We risk a great deal with our minor eating sins. Most of us are *not* constantly stuffing our faces and we have gained very little each year, but it has added up. In fact, most of us have been trying to reduce our body fat for many years, if not for several decades, but we fail because we don't understand or even know many of the basics explained in this book.

Most of us gain only a few to several grams per day and can barely notice it until our clothes get snug, and then we up-size our clothing one size after a few years to avoid the truth. But, as we all know, clothes sizes are not particularly consistent, so we blame it on clothing fit. Our fat gain puts our health at risk and we need to protect ourselves, so we end up fooling ourselves by getting great health and life insurance policies, imagining that somehow this will keep us healthy and alive. But nothing could be further from the truth. It's not wrong to have these insurances, but when we pretend as if they help us with our health, we are sorely mistaken.

These insurance policies are really improperly named; they should be called *disease* and *death* insurance, respectively. We can only use life insurance when we die, and as for health insurance, it is seldom used for making us healthier. Instead it is all too often used to hide our sins through expensive medications and analysis, expensive medications and analysis that we generally would not need if only we were at a healthy weight and would have taken good care of our bodies in the past.

We all need to understand that when we have the wrong perspective view of health and the health care industry, including medical care and insurances, we tend to depend upon others for our health. But in reality, they can do nothing for us regarding our health, except give advice and possibly alleviate some of our misery—but only temporarily. It is only each one of us that can heal ourselves and we do that with our own eating and internal health and mental protections.

Our bodies have many vital organs, but there are several that are very important to us regarding our weight. The first and most important is our brain and its mental condition. When we believe the wrong things, it is very bad for our health, and that is our first protection to be aware of and to address.

Keeping Heathy Kidneys

We also have physical protections in our vital organs and we must guard those protections very carefully if we want to be healthy and fit. Our kidneys are among those vital organs. Kidneys are located below our ribs on each side.

Healthy kidneys filter gallons of blood per hour. The filtration removes waste from our blood which is where our urine comes from. Our urine goes through tubes from our kidneys to our bladder and then the bladder holds the urine until we pee.

The waste and various acids are removed from our bodies by the filtration, allowing the body to keep a healthy balance of moisture and nutrients in our blood to be distributed to other parts of the body. If we don't take proper care of our kidneys, then our body chemistry will get out of balance and negatively affect our muscles, nerves, and other body parts, along with various hormones.

Without a healthy balance, our body cannot not work normally because our health negatively affects our nerves, muscles, and other tissues, and some the hormones that assist in controlling our red blood cell count and our blood pressure. The awesome kidneys transfer nutrients, fluids, and waste to the proper places for use, or for disposal via sweat and urine.

Our blood circulates through our kidneys quite a few times throughout the day to an amount that can exceed fifty gallons per day. If we damage this filter, or cause it to have to work harder by over consuming food and drink, then we risk damaging or substantially inhibiting the kidneys. Anytime we mess with our hormones in a negative way it will have negative effects on our quest to lose fat-weight.

Keeping a Healthy Liver

Located above the stomach on the left side and below our lungs, our livers are critical organs doing many important processes and are a part of the digestive system. The liver makes protein and breaks it down for digestion, it also detoxes and causes some digestive chemistry, and luckily for us and our bad eating habits, it is capable of some self-regeneration.

But when we push it to its limits by over-consuming something, such as is done with alcohol abuse, we then inhibit the liver's regeneration process, thus damaging the liver. Nutrient filled blood is sent to the liver from the digestive system along with oxygen filled blood from the heart. But when our digestive system is carrying too much toxic waste matter, it affects our blood and then that blood affects the liver.

The liver produces bile which allows the intestines to break down and absorb fats and some vitamins. Bile also helps in excreting waste when we sit on the toilet. Bile breaks down fat in our foods making them easier to digest. The liver also stores carbohydrates to be processed and converted into glucose, giving us stable blood-sugar levels. These sugars are then released when our bodies need quick energy.

The liver also filters and removes substances such as the hormone estrogen, along with substances that we consume such as alcohol or drugs. Keeping our livers healthy is critical because a damaged or poorly functioning liver is dangerous and all too often it can be fatal. Fatty liver disease commonly occurs when we are too fat or abuse alcohol.

When we eat too much fat, that fat can overwork the liver causing other functions of the liver to suffer. So when we have a poor functioning liver, it inhibits proper processing of the foods we eat causing us to *not* lose weight as desired.

Being fat, processing too much fat, excessive alcohol, and medications and drugs can negatively affect the liver, causing untold misery and frustration. And even though it is capable of regenerating itself, the liver needs to be reasonably healthy to regenerate, and regeneration takes time. The best way to keep your liver healthy is to make healthy food and drink choices in moderate quantities.

Keeping a Healthy Pancreas

A healthy pancreas creates the chemistry that is critical for proper digestion and fat loss. The insulin that the pancreas creates helps to stabilize blood sugar levels that, in turn, allow storage or use of the energy that is stored as fat in our bodies. With all that the pancreas does, it is easy to understand why keeping it healthy is so very important.

Keep that Heart Pumping

Let's not over-exert the heart either. The heart is perhaps the single most important organ in the body besides the brain. When we have fat build up around the heart, or in the main arteries, it slows our blood circulation and our heart has to then work even harder to pump the flow of blood throughout the body. When the blood cannot flow effectively, then the functions of the previously discussed organs also suffer. When all of these vital organs are negatively affected, we become very unhealthy and are greatly inhibited from losing the fat-weight that is causing our problems to begin with.

Our blood and the prompt and efficient circulation of that blood is vital. When the blood is not efficiently sent throughout the body, then the body and all of its organs and their functions will be deprived of the required nutrients that allow them all to function.

There is no need to over-exert ourselves or our hearts, but we should at least be doing enough activity on most days so that our hearts pumps well above our at-rest beat-rate for several minutes per day. But you must check with your doctor as to what activity levels are okay for you, because it is never worth dying due to improper exercise for any particular person's health condition.

The DreamThin Approach

The DreamThin approach is more about *understanding* than it is anything else. When we understand all of these vital organs and their unique functions, then we begin to understand how they can be so critical to our weight-loss efforts. In this chapter we merely lightly touched on just a few of our vital organs and their abilities. DreamThin is a self-motived discipline strategy that will change your bad habits to good ones if you are willing to understand and use sound logic in all you do regarding fat-weight loss.

Ease of DreamThin

I often hear people say that losing weight is too much work, but this is simply not true. Since the DreamThin approach doesn't suggest any additional exercises and only suggests considering accurate recording of all numbers and healthy and safe nutritionist-physician approved modification of eating habits, it is actually easier to do than it was to gain our fat-weight. To gain weight we must eat and chew, and chew, and chew. We have to get up and go and grab a snack or prepare the food we are about to abuse. But when using the DreamThin approach we do nothing and lose weight while sleeping and possibly even during the daytime hours. By not eating as much, and when taking a moment to record what we eat and the DreamThin Dollar value of that food, we can all DreamThin. It really is that easy!

How to Use DreamThin Checkbook Journal Pages

To an overweight person, not counting Calories is like a poor man not tracking how much he is spending when writing checks. It is very likely he will overdraw his checking account, thus creating a heavy load of unwanted and unneeded debt.

We must learn how to count calories until we fully understand just how much we're eating. Accurately recording our calorie consumption and burning off calories forces us to learn this basic skill. But doing so also tracks our progress so that we can make a reasonably accurate prediction as to when we will complete our personal perfect weight goal.

When using a DreamThin Checkbook Journal page as shown in the back of this book, you start with a balance owed to Fat & Co. and you then increase that balance when you eat, or you decrease the balance owed with your daily at rest payment and the payments made from additional activities. Remember: each calorie is equal to one penny.

Logging It

Log everything from the biggest burger to the smallest stick of gum. When we fail to log it, we tend to lie to ourselves about our actual calorie consumption. This quickly becomes a problem because many, if not most, of us are only over our daily needs by a relatively small amount and are adding only a few grams of fat per day to our waistline; so, when we imagine that we are "dieting", we are typically not when we fail to record everything. It is very easy to inaccurately estimate to the tune of a hundred or more calories per day. Unrecorded dieting often results in fat-weight gain rather than fat-weight loss, due to our failure to be true and accurate.

Your Debt and DreamThin Dollars

Each DreamThin Dollar is worth one hundred calories and will pay down the debt to Fat & Co. quickly when we understand and accurately record our calories. When we make our DreamThin Oath to ourselves and keep it, we will lose the unwanted fat on a consistent basis.

*When we are **honest** in our entries*, by the time our personal perfect weight has been achieved and the Fat & Co. debt is gone, that which weighs us down will also be gone–and that is your DreamThin Oath!

Chapter 10

Be Committed

When we make a DreamThin Oath to ourselves we must be committed to that Oath. When we fail in that commitment, we sabotage ourselves. Our commitment to our Oath keeps us focused allowing us to progress to our proper healthy fat-weight loss goal. When our progress is visible, it reinforces our resolve to stay committed to our own personal DreamThin Oath.

The best part is that once we understand some basic information about our bodies and the foods that we eat, then it's easier to lose fat-weight. And when that fat-weight loss truly begins, it gives us incentive to speed things up by adding a little more activity to our day. Every minute of exercise is roughly a nickel of payment to Fat & Co. A nickel doesn't sound like much, but a ten- to twenty-minute walk is worth around a fifty-cent reduction of your Fat & Co. balance that you owe. Do this a couple of times per day and at the end of the year you paid off an extra three-hundred-fifty dollars. These things do add up and they offer other health benefits as well!

Movement Matters

Movement is very important for fat-weight loss and also for good health. Exercise is fine to do, but that is not the kind of movement being referred to here. Many of our modern jobs require sitting still at a desk for hours on end. This stagnant posture is putting many of us in an early grave.

Though they are tightly connected, let's separate health issues from fat-loss issues. There are two critically important matters that help to keep us healthy: Getting proper nutrition, and getting enough movement. Nowhere is this more true than in our torso area. When we workout safely or have jobs that require a lot of torso movement, it is typically very good for our system. The torso movement makes our blood flow more freely because we are flexing the inner parts that are inside of our torso cavity and our heart rate increases as well. This increased blood flow greatly aids in processing our foods and removing impurities from our body and blood. If we consider that the organs spoken of in the last chapter are all in the torso area, it is easy to see how movement of the torso area can help those organs do their job more effectively.

It's great to get our limbs moving as well, but nothing will keep us healthier than proper and safe torso movement. Besides aiding in blood circulation, torso movement also helps our digestion and can alleviate issues surrounding the rate that our food passes through us, thus alleviating constipation. When food sits in our system too long it can cause untold problems. This is because as our bodies process the food, and as the food get closer and closer to exiting the body, the remaining waste becomes more and more toxic to us as the nutrients are all removed from that final material. If this toxic waste matter sits in us too long, then we tend to start feeling ill in various ways. Keeping a good flow of quality food passing through the system by eating well and getting enough torso movement keeps us healthier than we would otherwise be in a sedentary life style.

Exercise

When we don't have the luxury of a job that gives us lots of torso movement, then doing some simple and brief exercises that cause such movement can help us to live longer and have a better quality of life. Finding safe ways to get our torsos to twist and bend is usually a good idea after consulting with a physician about safe exercise for yourself.

But it's similar with our limbs. Our limbs are not as critical as our torso area, but blood flow to our limbs is what moves the fat stores both into and out of the body. When areas on the body suffer from low blood circulation, it inhibits the exchange of chemistry in those areas. This can result in modest variation in fat in the areas lacking proper circulation and can aid in the onset of other ailments such as some cancers or lumps.

Our bodies *need* circulation, and bad posture habits that are repetitive and occur for long durations, such as sitting on your foot all the while you watch TV in the evening, or crossing your legs a certain way while sitting at work can inhibit circulation to very specific areas on our bodies. When the circulation is cut off or is greatly reduced, then various toxins can build up in those areas causing us a great deal of perplexing pain along with unwanted expense in doctor bills. It is because we fail to connect our posture and activity levels to our health problems that our ailments perplex us. But when we realize that there are connections of our posture and movement to our health, then we can analyze our every move, allowing us to quickly come to realize that the little things we do can hurt us a lot.

While it is commonly referred to as "exercise", I prefer to refer to it as "movement". "Exercise" has become a dirty word for many of us who don't have much ambition, so calling it "movement" is better because simply getting the torso moving several times per day for several minutes can make a very big difference in our health. It can be from doing something around the house that you love to do, or it can be at your job, or it can be exercises. It really doesn't matter as long as you get the movement. Regarding constipation, getting torso movement has a similar effect on us as it does for the dog when taking the dog for a walk.

Activity and movement are good for our bodies as long as we don't overdo it or hurt ourselves in the process. If you have not been getting much movement, check with your nutritionist-physician or a professional trainer to find out what is best for you. They can help you think through your day-to-day meals and activity and then they can make recommendations as to your movement and eating needs.

Exercise Is a Bonus

Aside of the general movement activity just mentioned, exercise is a definite bonus regarding fat-weight loss. The choice is yours if you want to take advantage of that bonus. When it comes to fat loss, a little bit of exercise is like having a second job to help pay off your Fat & Co. debt more quickly. We will always benefit from exercise if we do it properly. Once our fat begins to subside and we see progress, it can be very exhilarating to do those extra exercises and watch the progress of our fat-weight loss speed up as the fat pounds melt away.

Take advantage of this bonus because it speeds up fat loss and keeps the blood circulating as well, thus benefitting your organs, your fat loss, your entire body, and your mind.

The Most Effective Way to Exercise

Exercise is a tough topic where it is best to not give recommendations because every situation and individual is unique. No one, except you and your nutritionist-physician, can really know what is best for you when it comes to exercise. Too often we are so eager to lose our fat that we over-do exercise and end up injured or even dead. It all depends on how well you know your own body, your health, and your abilities. Extreme workouts are usually not a particularly good idea and often end in injury.

It is said that the best way to exercise is to have a variety of exercises that you do and then do each in sets of five or ten repetitions. Let's say someone has ten different exercises they might do. They can pick about five and then do five to ten repetitions of each one until all are done and then do that five times over. But exercises are a somewhat personal matter and the person doing them must consider several things.

First, we must consider safety. If you feel, or your nutritionist-physician feels, that a certain exercise might cause you problems, then you are best to wait until you have conditioned yourself for such exercises and your nutritionist-physician okays it.

Next, we have to consider what our goals are with the exercises. Do we want to lose weight, or gain muscle? Are we trying to sculpt our bodies a bit and increase certain muscles like the highly sought after "six-pack-abs", or maybe lift the butt a bit? Or do we just want to tone up a bit and increase the biceps?

The most effective way to exercise will depend upon your goals. When wanting to lose fat, the task is often a multifaceted set of goals because we often want it all. If we are willing to work for it, we typically can have it all. A good time to begin sculpting your muscles through exercise is when you're planning to exercise anyway for the purpose of losing fat-weight, then you can burn up calories while sculpting the body.

But regardless of what we want to achieve, everyone must understand that muscle is wrongly believed to be far heavier than fat, but it is not. The two are very close in weight, yet a muscularly toned person who is the same weight and size as a non-toned person will usually look thinner. Additionally, when two people who are about the same size, a muscular toned person can be considerably heavier but look much thinner than the other person who is not muscular. This is because muscle has the ability to offer form, but fat does not. Muscle stays where we build and tone it, where fat, on the other hand, will sag, making us look heavier than we envisioned.

There are many types of exercises, and each of us must decide our own end goals and use the exercises as a means to achieve those goals. Depending upon your health condition and your goals, the exercises you personally choose will vary. Again, it is very important that you and your doctor understand your safe exercise levels. And then as you move forward, those exercises may be able to be increased if your physician says it is safe to do in order to achieve the levels that will speed up meeting your fat-weight-loss goals and reduce your fat even faster. Always work out safely with exercises that are safe for *you* after consulting with your nutritionist-physician.

Work It Through Your Body

Work it through the body. For instance, if you are doing stretches and you "feel the burn", also try something safe that is going to cause good overall blood circulation such as a few jumping jacks, torso twists, squats, or toe touches. The principle here is that acids forming that cause that burn need to be carried throughout your system via the circulation of your blood. The more fresh blood that we can circulate to any area helps the process of repairing muscles and reducing fat. The circulatory system has a specific purpose and when you understand it, then it becomes easier to use it safely to your own advantage. And nowhere is this more obvious than when trying to lose fat.

Different Kinds of Exercise

There are different kinds of exercise for different reasons. You can work out to build muscle but not lose any fat. But if you're not exercising enough, or more importantly you are not reducing your calorie intake, then the muscle you build will be buried in fat when you are over fat-weight. You could actually end up gaining weight because you are increasing muscle but not losing any fat. Generally, muscle-building targeted exercises will not burn much fat calories because most of those exercises don't work your entire system to circulate the blood as vigorously as exercises that increase your heart rate do. To burn a lot of calories your heart rate typically will need to noticeably increase to safe levels while you exercise.

What is Right for You

Know and understand the basics. If you don't care about building muscle, then exercise is not going to be important to you. Simply taking walks or jogging could be enough to help boost the fat removal. But, if you want to look more toned and not have saggy areas on your body when you're all done losing all of your unwanted fat, then something as simple as stretching exercises might be your thing. If you want muscular legs and "six-pack-abs" then you will have to do exercises such as squats, stomach-crunches and sit-ups. Deciding what is right for you will greatly depend upon your end goals and physical condition and discussions with your nutritionist-physician.

Main Exercise Considerations

- Exercise safely so that you do not injure yourself!
- When trying to lose the fat-weight, consider exercises that increase circulation.
- Understand the estimated number of calories you will burn and be accurate when recording those amounts.
- Understand what the various exercises do and how and why they can benefit you and your goals.
- Choose the right exercises for you and your goals.
- Understand that exercise burns less calories than we want to imagine.

- Understand how many calories a single bite of something actually has, because single bite of some foods after workout can easily cause the need for an additional fifteen minutes of workout time, where the original workout time, on the other hand, was intended to offset what you have previously eaten.

Jogging four miles in about an hour might burn up roughly three hundred calories. But popping a seventy-five-calorie cookie into your mouth will sabotage fifteen to twenty minutes of that hour-long jog. There is a list shown in a following chapter that demonstrates the cost to our waistline when various foods are put in our mouths, along with what we need to do to pay off the Fat & Co. debt that those foods cost us.

Chapter 11

You Receive what You Eat

Eating is one of the few pleasures that we all can enjoy, but we all enjoy it a little too much. Our culturally-increasing waistlines have been blamed on our culturally-increasingly sedentary desk jobs. But at the same time that our computers entered the scene, so did an onslaught of convenience food that all of us are all too happy to have in the office or at our desks. And especially if we have desk jobs, our access to high-calorie foods and meals has been increased so much that it is almost impossible to not cross paths with these foods many times throughout the day.

If we consume more calories than we need for the body's activity level, then we will receive what we eat in the form of added fat.

Hunger

"Hunger" is mostly in the head. If you really want to lose your fat weight then you must learn to deal with the sensation of "hunger pains". In truth, there are very few people in the developed world who really know hunger. Most of us feel the rumbling of digestion and believe it to be hunger pains. But that is not real hunger. We are well-fed, too well-fed in fact, which is why we are getting fat.

When we reduce our eating quantities and clear our system then we will most likely experience those rumbles that we all know can be quieted by eating. The problem with this is that too often we eat enough for an entire meal when this happens, when nothing more than a small bite or a small piece of sucking candy can stop it. In fact, nothing more than just smelling food can sometimes stop the rumbling, but smelling food can also cause rumbling to begin.

When our system has been cleared and we eat in proper and healthy ways regarding the quantity eaten at each sitting, then the rumbling usually gets better and occurs less often, if at all. Don't be fooled by noisy digestion. When in doubt, consult with your nutritionist-physician.

Find what works best for you to stop you from consuming too much when those rumbles occur, because those rumbles sabotage the efforts of many people. But beside the rumbles in our digestive system we also have "cravings".

Mining for Food

Once we eliminate the myth that some foods are bad, we can get on to truly understanding all foods. Food is food, including all drinks. But different foods do have different nutritional value. It is the nutritional value, or lack thereof, that gives some foods a bad reputation. But these negative attitudes towards low nutritional value foods are unfair to those foods. If low-nutrition "junk foods" were being portrayed as high-nutrition foods that would be different, but they are being portrayed as snack and party foods. And trying to compare them to meal foods is somewhat of an idiotic and unfair approach.

These foods are enjoyable for us, and provided that we eat them in *reasonable quantities*, they generally won't harm us, and they can actually benefit us if they make us feel some joy, as long as we don't overdo it and abuse them. Remember, even water can harm us when we drink too much.

The problem we have is that, as mentioned earlier in the book, we eat too much of those foods that have low nutritional value and we eat too little of the foods with high nutritional value. It is not the food's fault, it is our own fault.

Here is the problem when we over-eat snack foods and under-eat high-nutrition foods: Our bodies need, desire, and crave nutrition. Those odd cravings that we have are often for foods that contain the needed vitamins and minerals that we are actually craving. But when our bodies are accustomed to eating large quantities of low-nutrition foods, then our bodies will seek the desired nutrition from the low-nutrition foods. And because those foods lack a great deal regarding a particular point of nutrition, the particular nutritional cravings won't cease as we would like them to. This is often misunderstood by us as cravings for the specific food, when generally it is a craving for the nutrients we lack. And as long as we are short on those nutrients, our craving will likely continue, causing us to overeat all the more.

Let's say that you're mining for gold and you are in a low gold content area, then you will have to sift through a lot more dirt in order to find enough gold to make it worth your while doing the work. But if you are in an area with a high concentration of gold then you don't have to work very hard to find lots of gold. That is exactly how food is and the low-nutritional value foods are like the areas with very low concentrations of gold.

Nutrients are gold for our bodies and when our food lacks those nutrients then the body must process much more food in order to find enough food-gold in the form of nutrients to keep our bodies whole and healthy. When the systems of the body are forced to dig through so much more food to find a few scant bits of nutritional gold, then we are also processing many more calories, and many of those calories will be stored as fat. To assist in reducing cravings for low-nutrition food, make sure to get enough high nutritional value foods to meet your daily nutrition needs.

Also, when we lack nutrition, our digestive system is going to do its best to extract the nutrients from the food in our digestive system, and that can slow down the food passing through us. Eating proper amounts of high-nutrition food is very important to your health!

Eat Balanced Meals

The fundamental principle of DreamThin is that when we eat right and we make sure we eat at a frequency so as to have our bodies be able to burn off some fat between meals, especially while we sleep, the fat will be slowly reduced on a daily basis until we reach equilibrium or until we have met our goal. And when our calorie consumption is lower than our calorie usage, our weight will drop until we achieve our safe personal perfect weight, at which point we can slowly increase our daily calorie intake until we stop losing fat or until we begin to gain weight again. At that time, we adjust to a point where our weight remains stable.

It doesn't much matter what we eat, even if it is junk food, because we can still lose weight eating only junk food. But eating *only* junk food is not ever recommended because our bodies suffer a great deal because of the critical nutrition we miss by failing to eat high-nutrient foods.

Whether we want to believe it or not, our bodies want good food and need it. Eating fruits, veggies, meat, dairy, bread, and cereals in the proper quantities will help us lose weight faster than if all we eat is always only chips and soda. We also have to consider quality of life. Often when we overdo it on low-nutrient foods, our health suffers and we end up with indigestion and all sorts of other health ailments.

If we only knew what a difference eating enough foods with proper nutrients can make regarding our health, then most of us would quickly make the adjustment in eating habits and be able to reduce expensive doctor visits and medications pertaining to the ailments caused by lack of proper nutrition. This is not a small problem in our culture–it is an epidemic! It is not so much *what* we are eating as it is what we are ***not*** eating that causes our health problems.

Balanced eating habits have been, are now, and will always be the best for our bodies. "Balanced meals" has come to mean that we have food from certain food groups, and this is true. But a truly balanced meal is one that supplies enough of each nutrient so that at the end of each day you have consumed enough of each nutrient required for your body to stay healthy and in full functioning order.

When our bodies are not properly nutrified, it can inhibit our ability to lose fat and it typically diminishes our health and causes a great deal of seemingly unexplainable symptoms. These symptoms often get misdiagnosed as one disease or another. It's amazing what a difference proper nutrition can make to our cravings, to our health, and to our quest to permanently rid ourselves of excess fat.

Understanding What to Eat

Earlier in this book, we discussed how all foods are demonized by someone somewhere at some point. One person says dairy is bad, another says fruit is bad, and another says veggies are bad, etc. Who should we believe? Probably none of them. All foods are good and are nothing more or less than food, but they do have varying nutritional content and that is what we need to grasp.

It typically doesn't matter what you eat as long as you are consuming your daily nutritional needs and not consuming too many calories.

A wide variety of food tends to be the most effective at keeping us healthy. When our health is ailing from some disease or condition, then seeking additional high-nutrition foods recommended by a nutritionist-physician may be of some help for most people when the nutrition is aimed at the needs for combating the specific disease or condition.

Eat what suits you and gives you the nutrients required for your body to be healthy and will not cause you to consume too many calories when working to lose the fat you want to lose.

Understanding How to Eat

Eating is eating, right? Not exactly. Our culture has done a great job at advertising gluttony, and that is the one major sin of the food industry. There is nothing wrong with any food, it is the quantity of those foods consumed that harms us. But here, when understanding *how* to eat, we are not referring to how much to eat, but rather how to actually eat it.

When we eat, we are encouraged by advertisers to consume, telling us to "guzzle it" and "chomp it", thus encouraging extra consumption. We can't really blame them for this because that's how they earn their money. It's our own fault for following such foolish suggestions. We can consume those products, but it is up to us to moderate the quantity that we consume and the frequency at which we do so.

What we really need to do is to eat in moderation and chew, chew, chew our food. When we chew our foods very well, it better satisfies our hunger and cravings because our system is then able to more quickly extract the needed nutrients from the food. This allows us to feel full faster and longer. And it is our feeling of being satisfied longer that stops us from craving more food sooner.

The time we spend eating can and should be a time of joy, and we should take our time and chew well and then give the meal time to do its work. But when we guzzle and chomp it all down too quickly, we end up eating more than needed because the needed nutrients have not been able to penetrate our system quickly enough, thus leaving us feeling unfulfilled.

When food is chewed well and then swallowed, it helps the digestion considerably and aids in reducing indigestion. When we fail to completely chew our foods, the larger pieces of that food sit within the stomach. It takes more time for the acidic digestion process to break down the larger chucks of food. Think of it in terms of ice melting in a drink. If the ice cubes are smaller chunks then the pieces melt quickly, but if the ice is made of large cubes then it takes longer for each piece to completely melt. It is much the same with food, except the food is not melting, it is being broken down and dissolved by stomach acids. This can occur more rapidly when we chew well and crush and grind the food into finer pieces with our teeth. If we all did this, it would help all of us better extract the needed nutrients and deliver them more quickly and efficiently to the entire system.

If we fail to properly masticate (masticate is to chew), then we don't always get the full benefit from the foods. If food goes through our system in a partially undigested form, then we missed out on the nutrition that we could have gained from that food.

Chewing foods well can often reduce or eliminate indigestion, reduce chances of choking on the food, increase absorption of nutrients, make us feel full more quickly and for longer periods of time. There really is no downside to thoroughly chewing your food.

Understand When to Eat

With regard to losing fat, understanding when to eat is not really important, but understanding when *not* to eat is. Only you can decide for yourself *when* you should eat and *what* you should eat. All that anyone else can do is offer information so that you can make great decisions for yourself!

When trying to lose fat and get your body down to a healthy fat-weight, and keep it there, you need to know that you have three choices to lose weight in a healthy way. You do so by eating less, or exercising, or you do both.

When trying to lose weight by exercising, we must understand that we have to exercise a lot to use enough calories to compensate enough for our over-indulgence in food. A half cup of ice cream takes roughly a four mile walk to burn off those calories, and that depends upon your height, gender, and size. A petite female will have to walk considerably longer than a six-foot-two fully grown man in order to burn the same number of calories that the ice cream had.

To effectively lose weight without exercise, there must reliably be periods during a 24-hour day that you don't eat anything so that your body can get into the fat burning mode. The best time to do this is a night while sleeping. If we fill up late at night shortly before bed, it presents problems for our system. The first problem is that since we will soon be lying down in bed, our body is not moving and can't move the food through our system as quickly as it otherwise would. And our blood circulation is reduced when at rest, thus causing our digestion to slow down. Then as our system breaks the foods down, those foods will sit nearly stagnant in our stomach because we are not moving, which is a major cause of acid reflux or indigestion.

And regarding weight, the worst part about eating late is that since we just fueled up and our digestion will slow down slightly because we're not moving, the energy from the food, measured in calories, will slowly be extracted *all night long.* This is not a problem in itself, but it is when trying to lose fat-weight.

Eating shortly before bed works similar to sipping on a large soda or sugar laden latte all day long. The calories from the food eaten just before bed will be used for your basic at rest sustenance, thus stopping your body from achieving a fat-burning state while you sleep.

Those of us whose eating is pretty good and our calories are close to where they belong, but we can't seem to lose the fat, might begin to lose fat by eating earlier and getting some mild exercise after our last meal and/or last snack for the evening, but well before we go to bed for the night The concept is that we must, at some point, short our bodies the calories that it uses to function so that it has an opportunity to draw from our massive fat stores. It is only when our body taps into those fat stores that we will actually lose fat-weight. Tapping into the fat stores of our body is the only way we lose fat and **there is no other way.** So, either we exercise or we cut calories, or we do both. But knowing when *not* to eat can speed things up. And depending upon your current eating habits, changing *when* you eat can allow those whose intake is proper and who are trying to lose fat-weight to do so *with nothing more than changing* ***when*** you eat.

After consulting with your nutritionist-physician, take in only the number of calories that allows you to burn fat during the time between meals, including, and especially, the time from supper- and night-time snack until breakfast.

Chapter 12

Your Guide to Success

We often seek out multi-step programs, telling us to do this, and then that, with each step having a specific instruction. But if we want to attack this fat-weight problem and properly deal with it, then our best guide to success is going to be knowledge, and more importantly *understanding* of that knowledge. Just because we can recite chapter and verse of a medical journal does not mean that we *understand* it.

The world is full of good books and weight loss programs with steps to do this and steps to do that, but there are really only two steps. First you must understand and second you must implement that understanding. If you don't cut your calories, or in some other way cause a calorie deficit, it is impossible to lose the fat. Exercise isn't exactly cutting calories, but it does accomplish the same thing; exercise causes the body to be short of calories needed, causing a calorie deficit, thus allowing your body to begin to use the energy stored as fat that hangs around the waistline and other parts of the body.

Let proper understanding be your guide to success, rather than worn-out old seven-step programs that have not been working for you.

Real Life is Not Soundbites from Commercials

Every form of media is desperately trying to get your attention. This is why many news headlines are really quite stupid, because they prey on our sense of curiosity. The more outrageous they can make things sound, then the more articles we tend to read, ending with us seeing more advertising which pays the salaries of the news people. The same effect is true with weight loss. Clever sayings and short catchy tidbits grab our attention as they are intended to, and catch our attention is all they really do.

We read ads in magazines, we see ads on TV, we listen to ads on the radio, and most, if not all of them, will have some catchy alluring hook to get our attention. There's nothing wrong with this, but too often *we* waste our time and money on vague promises only to fail time and time again. We fail because when we are told that we can lose ten pounds in seven days, we miss the part that says "up to" ten pounds. And more importantly, we miss the part that says "when you follow our program" which is the part that actually causes you to lose actual fat, following what ends up being basic biophysics.

If you're the type to get sucked in by the soundbites, then make sure you pay attention to the fine print, because it is going to tell you that you must exercise and/or eat right. Everything else about the program is advertising hype to get us to buy the program.

There is no weight loss program, and their never will be one, that will allow us to eat whatever we want and as much as we want and not exercise and also lose fat at the same time. We can lose weight, and we might be able to eat our favorite foods in large quantities without reserve or hesitation, but there will always be a catch somewhere in the plan that allows for the body to regularly enter into a calorie deficit position in regard to calories-in versus calories-out. And it is only a calorie deficit that allows us to burn off the fat. We **must** be in a calorie deficit position long enough so that there are more calories burned than are being absorbed during the non-deficit periods of the day. This is a simple scientific truth and it applies to anyone who has ever lived, or who is alive now, or who will be born in the future. This simple scientific fact cannot be thwarted. It is just the way the body works.

You are far better off when you have a clear grasp of food and of your body. And when you understand how the functions of energy-used versus energy-consumed works, then it is far easier to lose the fat while also having a robust and diverse food selection that allows you to eat whatever you want. The catch is that you cannot eat as *much* as you want anytime you want it without any exercise.

Battle of College Obesity

If you're a college student, or are the parent of a college student, learn early that eating chips and pizza all night while studying is a one-way ticket to being fat. The waist sizes of students today are increasing at an ever-alarming rate. And with all of the "studying" going on, it is only going to get worse. If we are sedentary during study, and then party afterwards consuming snacks and/or alcohol, then we are pretty much guaranteed to get fat.

There was a time when fat gain was relegated mostly to wealthy older men and women who did not have particularly active lives and who also had abundant food at their every whim. But with our current social affinity towards convenience and snack foods, nearly everyone can readily afford to have their eating outpace their body's ability to burn off the excess energy.

We all need to understand the following, from this moment forward if we want to avoid fat in our future: A typical average woman needs approximately 1,375 calories per day. And a typical average man needs approximately 1,650 calories per day. If you are taller than average or shorter than average or if you are very active then these average numbers will increase or reduce accordingly. Nothing is going to change this basic fact. There is no miracle for fat reduction except for the truth, and the truth requires that we alter our eating and/or activity to a point of calorie deficit in order to lose weight. If you are very active then you can eat more and not gain weight.

Beware of Bad Information

Many paper and electronic publications have jumped on the weight-loss bandwagon and simply repeat things other people say, without mathematically checking the facts.

A big part of the problem is our interpretation of the government information on food consumption. The U.S. government uses broad statements and averages to address well over 300 million people and it also quotes medical journals, all of which is okay. But when interpreted, we often take the high number and use it as our own personal index. We believe things like if you're a female then your body should not exceed 30% fat or you will be obese, but at 29.999% you're not obese. Is this reality? No, reality is that a female should be between about 10% to 25% body fat but near 18% to 20% is the actual target. The 30% is the breakpoint where we are forced to admit that we have become fat. It's not that we didn't notice this at 29.999% fat, but rather we just choose to close our eyes to the truth as long as we are able.

Things are not much different regarding our perception of fat in foods. Make no mistake about it, proper fat is good and it is needed for your body to properly function. But why do we put protein at 10% to 15% of our daily calories and carbohydrates at

50% to 60% and fat squarely at 30%, why not 15% to 30%? It is said that if you are exceeding 30% fat consumption that you are then consuming too much fat. We need to realize that when simple points like this get missed, it causes big problems in our thinking because we look at these government *guidelines* as *requirements* rather than *the maximum daily limit* that these numbers are typically conveying.

Regarding the Nutrition Facts on food labels, the important part is the amount of nutrients we get from the food and the overall calories for the amount we are consuming. Unless you have some serious health condition, the fat, protein, and carbohydrate balance in the food is not particularly important because we typically eat enough different foods to supply our needs. Also remember that while we humans are very different than animals, what we are made of is very much the same. Just as a cow can live on mostly grass, humans also can live mostly on vegetables that have little if any fat. As mentioned in an earlier chapter, the body has the most amazing organs that can turn the foods we eat in to the needed fat, muscle, and bone. We tend to be healthier when we eat diverse foods rather than only vegetables, but the human body can survive on vegetables just like animals do.

It is common though for people who eat only vegetables to have vitamin deficiencies and they typically need to take supplements in that case. But when you have proper healthy and diverse eating habits, you then typically need not take supplements and will have a well-functioning body that looks good and is fit and trim.

Be Knowledgeable and Understand

Be knowledgeable about your fat-weight loss before you discuss it with others or all too often they will assume you will become anorexic on your way down that fat ladder, thus serving to undermine your mental disposition and your efforts. It is common that when your friends, family, and co-workers see you losing weight that they will often make foolish comments like "You're losing too much weight." Seldom is this true. Those around us are so accustomed to the way we have looked for so many years that it is somewhat alarming to them when we begin to get our fat-weight under control. Plus others may comment negatively out of sheer envy.

Clearly understand your proper personal perfect weight. When we have this well in mind when people say foolish things, we can either ignore it or tell them our healthy weight goal. When we are light on knowledge and understanding then when people say foolish things to us it greatly affects us because we are uncertain of our information and are likely to believe their ignorant statements. But when we *know* and *understand* what and why, then we can confidently achieve our goals *knowing* and *understanding* that we are doing it right with a healthy approach.

The Good News

The good news is that while we may have gained fat over many years, the majority of people can safely, effectively, and permanently use the fat to fuel the body. And depending on how much fat-weight we have, most of us can typically reduce our fat to healthy levels in less than a year. The concept of dreaming thin has safe goals and habits as a top priority. Those of us whose bodies have larger quantities of fat will need more time to reduce all of the excess body fat.

Losing a pound every week or two is reasonably easy to do for an average height adult. This means that since most people are only about fifty to a hundred pounds overweight, the fat that took so many years to accumulate can be safely gone in a year or two.

Some people choose extreme weight-loss programs, but those are not recommended due to increased possibility of injury or even death. Also, if you depend upon exercise alone to lose weight, then the moment you stop your exercise routines the weight will begin to come back again, and usually more aggressively than it did the first time.

Why DreamThin Works

Your personalized daily calorie reductions allow you to eat anything you want as long as your proper nutrition needs are being met. The catch on this is that you cannot eat as much as you had been eating in the past. Dreaming thin causes you to lose weight while sleeping, and will cause you to lose still more during active awake-hours without additional exercise when your body is in its calorie-deficit mode.

Among the many weight-loss programs in the marketplace, there are many good ones that work well when you stick to them. But there is an ignored reality that many of the weight-loss programs have closed their eyes to, which is that most of us actually need fewer calories than is typically recommended.

Because we love to eat, we look at these recommendations in a very rough manner using the national nutritional label figures as if they were specifically designed for each one of us personally. But they are not designed for us personally. Those facts and figures are put in a 2000-calorie index so that we have something to go by. It would be mathematically easier if they had used a 1000-calorie index or even a 100-calorie index. But the problem is that when the index is too small then the decimals used would be preceded by more zeros, nullifying their value to many minds. 2000 is a good number because it is close to the needs for an average *active* adult.

But when we misunderstand this 2000 calorie index and its purpose, then not only do we see it as a valid number for ourselves, but we also exceed it because we underestimate the calorie value of the foods we consume, thus causing us to get fat.

The DreamThin concept is to reveal truth. Your personal figures and calculations should be based upon *you*, *your* weight, *your* height, and *your* gender. Once we hit adulthood, age has little to do with our calorie needs. Some charts will show several frame sizes, but have unrealistic weights, especially for women. A big problem with our perception of how much people should weigh is that we often view *facts* incorrectly. For instance, the average weight in the 1960's of a 5 foot 4 inch female was about 135 lbs. That is the "average", not the "best" weight. The "average" 5 foot 4 inch woman today weighs about 160 lbs. The only thing here that changed, besides the weight of the "average", is the amount and type of calories that this average 5 foot 4 inch woman consumes. The reality is that if she is 5 feet 4 inches tall then her personal perfect weight is roughly about 115 pounds plus or minus about 8 pounds. And maybe add up to 10% to the high end if you're muscular.

Whether or not we eat small amounts often throughout the day instead of having a couple of meals has to be determined by each one of us based upon what works best for our own lifestyle. But when we nibble on food all throughout the day, we are rarely able to achieve the all-important state of calorie deficit.

When we nibble all day long, rather than having a few specific meals during the day, then making sure that we will be in calorie deficit while we sleep is critical. Otherwise there will be no time period during a 24-hour day that allows the body to enter into the fat burning mode long enough to actually lose your unwanted fat. We can nibble all day long if the hourly nibbling of calories does not exceed the hourly calories burned and still lose or maintain our weight. Successful, permanent, proper weight loss always and only comes from absorbing less calories, and the best tried and true way to do that is to... you guessed it, eat less! If you sleep eight hours, an average height woman will burn about 260 calories during the night, and an average height man will burn about 400 calories during the night. At 3500 calories per pound that is about 13 nights of sleep for an average height woman to lose 1 pound and 9 nights of sleep for an average height for man to lose one pound of fat-weight. Not a bad workout value for sleeping! Do nothing more than this for a year and the woman will have lost about 28 pounds and the man will have lost about 40 pounds by *sleeping*! Yes, SLEEPING!

In our quest to take shortcuts, especially in cases of extreme obesity, people will sometimes opt for gastric bypass surgery. Besides being dangerous, gastric bypass surgery will also fail if you manage to eat enough of the wrong foods after the vital parts of your intestines have been permanently removed and the surgery has healed. A less intrusive surgery option is liposuction; but liposuction is not permanent. Other than surgical removal of body fat, all surgery and/or diets ultimately cause the body to absorb less calories than it is using which can be done for free by changing some basic eating and activity habits.

What we eat does make a difference. For an average height adult female, properly balanced good eating habits of consuming approximately 1,375 calories per day will properly maintain your healthy weight. For average height adult males, it is approximately 1,650 calories. But the same calorie consumption with the wrong foods could cause the same person to slowly gain weight.

That old adage "You are what you eat" applies here. Some foods process more slowly than others. For instance, sugar in soda-pop will get into your system very quickly. Where pasta is somewhat slower and will give you energy for a longer period of time. Then there are items like protein from meat that takes very long to digest and absorb and some of it never completely breaks down and may get passed through only partially digested. When we eat foods that process quickly, then the body will heat up in effort to use that energy, but there are limits to that and some of the unused energy will be stored as fat.

When people choose to do very low carbohydrate diets, the principle is that when digesting, the fast-acting carbohydrates are then missing, thus the body is then forced to survive on proteins and fats. But the system cannot process protein and fat quickly enough to meet the body's calorie needs, so we end up burning off body fat. When using this very low carbohydrate method, according to the diet, we can consume as much protein and fat as we want and still lose weight, but that can very quickly become boring, and for some people doing so can be dangerous to their health.

Food is a tool that can be a joy when it is used properly, and a weapon when it is used improperly. And when we understand it as the tool that it is, then it is much easier to enjoy it guilt free because when we understand how to use that tool, we can manipulate our habits to our own best advantage. We do this by eating for the purpose of energy, nutrition, and clear thinking when needed, and we don't eat at certain times when we want to DreamThin.

Food Rule of Thumb

There really is no particular best way to know how many calories you are about to consume other than carrying a calorie book with you or accessing some lookup tool. But when all else fails, we can use generalizations to at least get us closer than what we do by blindly guessing at calorie content. Following are a few basic generalized categories that we can use as a very rough index when we have no other source of information at the time we are making our food selections. The following are listed in weight ounces:

- Sweet bakery donuts, cookies, etc. 120 Calories per ounce.
- Standard bakery bread, buns, etc. 70 calories per ounce.
- Regular Soda about 15 calories per ounce.
- Fruit is about 25 calories per ounce.
- Vegetables are about 25 calories per ounce.
- Butter and other fats are about 202 calories per ounce.
- Meats are about 100 calories per ounce.

The problem with such a simple rule of thumb is that the figures change greatly depending upon many factors. Some fruits and vegetables contain far greater amounts of water and therefore will be lower in calories than fruits and vegetables that have very low water content. Meat is a bit different because moisture is not as much of a factor as is fat content. Butter is mostly fat, and fat is very high in calories which is why we are required to use so much energy to lose a pound of our own body fat.

Since fat is very high in calories, the fat content of meat will increase or reduce the amount of calories in the meat we choose to eat. The same is true with baked goods regarding both fats and moisture.

Use generalized "Rules of Thumb" only as rough guides. Never depend on them for constant use. These sorts of indexes are for those times when we have nothing else to use as an index for tracking the calories we are about to consume.

Most people enjoy a treat now and then; so, following is a brief list showing calorie cost along with how much Fat & Co. will charge you for some of the snacks you might place into our mouth. Notice the amount of work required to pay back the calorie debt with something as small as a single tiny piece of chocolate candy–that we typically eat by the handful. That means that ten tiny chocolate candies will cost you 40 cents in additional debt to Fat & Co. And when you consider that those are chewed and swallowed in a matter of seconds, it brings a whole new awareness to the subject. Pay close attention to the following list because it contains the secret to most people's increased waistline:

Female (5 feet 4 inches) Eating Exercise Cost in Hours:Mins						
Snack	Desc	Calories	Fat Co	Walk	Run	SitUps
01 M&M (Plain)	1 Piece	4.3	$0.04	:02	:01	:03
02 Tootsie Pop	1 Lollypop	60	$0.60	:33	:12	:40
03 Doritos	1 Chip	14	$0.14	:08	:03	:09
04 Lay's (Original)	1 Chip	7.5	$0.08	:04	:02	:05
05 Oreo (Double)	1 Cookie	70	$0.70	:39	:15	:47
06 Cheetos (Puffs)	1 Cheeto	5.5	$0.06	:03	:01	:04
07 Hershey's Kiss	1 Kiss	25.5	$0.26	:14	:05	:17
08 Candy Corn	1 Piece	6.4	$0.06	:04	:01	:04
09 Candy Hearts	1 Piece	3.9	$0.04	:02	:01	:03
10 Wrigley's Gum	1 Stick	10	$0.10	:06	:02	:07
11 Pretzels	1 Pretzel	12.2	$0.12	:07	:03	:08

Male (5 feet 10 inches) Eating Exercise Cost in Hours:Mins						
Snack	Desc	Calories	Fat Co	Walk	Run	SitUps
01 M&M (Plain)	1 Piece	4.3	$0.04	:02	:01	:02
02 Tootsie Pop	1 Lollypop	60	$0.60	:21	:08	:21
03 Doritos	1 Chip	14	$0.14	:05	:02	:05
04 Lay's (Original)	1 Chip	7.5	$0.08	:03	:01	:03
05 Oreo (Double)	1 Cookie	70	$0.70	:25	:09	:25
06 Cheetos (Puffs)	1 Cheeto	5.5	$0.06	:02	:01	:02
07 Hershey's Kiss	1 Kiss	25.5	$0.26	:09	:03	:09
08 Candy Corn	1 Piece	6.4	$0.06	:02	:01	:02
09 Candy Hearts	1 Piece	3.9	$0.04	:01	:01	:01
10 Wrigley's Gum	1 Stick	10	$0.10	:04	:01	:04
11 Pretzels	1 Pretzel	12.2	$0.12	:04	:02	:04

Exercise Rule of Thumb

Since every person is built differently and has differing movement habits, a generalized chart can only roughly estimate how many calories a body might burn when doing certain activities. And because it is different for each person, it would fill several books to do a comprehensive listing. So what we have done here is to offer some basic median values for female and male. However, since the muscle mass for any particular person can vary a great deal, there is simply no way of knowing without in-person analysis even if the gender and height are known. As you view the list, consider how many minutes you must do the activity to compensate for the ten chocolate candies or 40 calories you might have eaten in only a few second's time.

Male (5 feet 10 inches) Rough Estimate Calories Burned				
Activity	**1-Min**	**15-Min**	**30-Min**	**1-Hour**
Aerobics, Basic	4.7	70	140	280
Automobile repair	2.8	42	84	168
Baby Stroller, pushing	2.3	35	70	140
Ballet Dancing	4.5	67	134	269
Construction, general	5.1	77	154	308
Football tackle	8.4	126	252	504
Gardening, general	3.7	56	112	224
Ice Skating general	6.5	98	196	392
Jogging, general	6.5	98	196	392
Jumping Rope	7.5	112	224	448
Mountain Biking	7.9	119	238	476
PC Work (typing)	1.4	21	42	84
Pushups, vigorous	7.5	112	224	448
Race Walking	6.1	91	182	364
Reading reclining	0.9	14	28	56
Running 5 Miles per hour	7.5	112	224	448
Running up stairs	14.0	210	420	840
Sewing, domestic	1.4	21	42	84
Soccer casual	6.5	98	196	392
Softball, general	4.7	70	140	280
Standing moderate work	3.3	49	98	196
Stretching	2.3	35	70	140
Swimming, general (leisure, not laps)	5.6	84	168	336
Tae Bo, moderate	11.2	168	336	672
Tennis, general	6.5	98	196	392
Trampoline	3.3	49	98	196
TV watching	0.9	14	28	56
Walking 3 miles per hour	3.1	46	92	185

Female (5 feet 4 inches) Rough Estimate Calories Burned				
Activity	1-Min	15-Min	30-Min	1-Hour
Aerobics, Basic	3.0	45	90	180
Automobile repair	1.8	27	54	108
Baby Stroller, pushing	1.5	23	45	90
Ballet Dancing	2.9	43	86	173
Construction, general	3.3	50	99	198
Football tackle	5.4	81	162	324
Gardening, general	2.4	36	72	144
Ice Skating, general	4.2	63	126	252
Jogging, general	4.2	63	126	252
Jumping Rope	4.8	72	144	288
Mountain Biking	5.1	77	153	306
PC Work (typing)	0.9	14	27	54
Pushups, vigorous	4.8	72	144	288
Race Walking	3.9	59	117	234
Reading reclining	0.6	9	18	36
Running 5 Miles per hour	4.8	72	144	288
Running up stairs	9.0	135	270	540
Sewing, domestic	0.9	14	27	54
Soccer casual	4.2	63	126	252
Softball, general	3.0	45	90	180
Standing moderate work	2.1	32	63	126
Stretching	1.5	23	45	90
Swimming, general (leisure, not laps)	3.6	54	108	216
Tae Bo, moderate	7.2	108	216	432
Tennis, general	4.2	63	126	252
Trampoline	2.1	32	63	126
TV watching	0.6	9	18	36
Walking 3 miles per hour	2.0	30	59	119

Handy Measure Volume Conversion

For home kitchen purposes, liquids are the same in weight ounces as they are in volume or liquid ounces. A cup, which is eight ounces of water, weighs about eight ounces on a scale, as do most other consumable liquids. However, powdered items such as flour and powder sugar have more volume ounces than they do weight ounces for a given ounce value. And it is very important that you understand that difference. The following indexes are all volume to volume conversions except for the last item on the list which is a weight to weight conversion.

16 cups = 1 gallon
8 pints = 1 gallon
4 quarts = 1 gallon
128 ounces = 1 gallon
3 3/4 liters(approx) = 1 gallon

8 ounces = 1 cup
16 Tablespoons = 1 cup
48 teaspoons = 1 cup
1/4 liter (approx) = 1 cup

2 Tablespoons = 1 ounce
6 teaspoons = 1 ounce
28 grams (approx) = 1 ounce

Chapter 13

There Are Many

We discussed some of the costs of being overweight in an earlier chapter, but let's revisit this with a bit more of a specific approach. Being over fat-weight has many hidden costs to all of us, ranging from making it harder to get a job, especially when the economy is not doing particularly well, to our health. A typical cost is the medical expenses we incur due to our own fat-weight problems. But there are other true hidden costs too. One is that our insurances are more expensive because so many of us are overextending our insurance privileges. And even if you are not buying your own insurance, then your employer probably is, and the extra expense they pay in insurance for you, cuts into what would otherwise have been a substantial raise in pay for you. Yet this is not the true hidden cost.

The true hidden cost to ourselves is our own quality of life and the allure of blaming our problems on everything but ourselves, thus barring us from ever being able to correct the problem. This problem negatively affects our lives and might put us in an early grave, even after spending all of that money on health insurance, medicine, and doctors.

Pharma Ads

Some of the advertisements for the pharmaceutical companies over the years have been very deceptive in portraying who is actually suffering from the symptoms the drugs are supposed to remedy.

The first major point is that very few of the prescription drugs on the market actually cure the underlying problem, because the drugs are generally designed to help us to feel less discomfort or aid in some aspect of our problems. These pharmaceutical companies are not in error in this regard; rather the error is in our misperception that we can be cured with these drugs.

The second point is that many of the pharmaceutical advertisements show very healthy-looking people who are actors and actresses who *probably don't use*, and likely never have used, the medications for which they appear in the ads. There is a reality, and that reality is that the majority of us who consume many of the pharmaceuticals on the market today are doing so because of our fat related health problems.

They don't talk about our fat problem in the ads and they tend to show healthy people because it's more appealing to all of us when they don't show the truth. We tend to listen more carefully and be more easily influenced when an advertisement is attractive to us. The imagery used helps to take away from the horrendous pharmaceutical side-effects that sometimes occur in people, which they usually read very quickly and/or show in fine print while the advertisement is shown. When we are over fat-weight then we can be pretty sure that many of these ads are intended for us. But the ads are for the side-effect of being overweight, such as type-two diabetes, or heart issues, sleep apnea, etc. rather than dealing with the real problem of us being way over fat-weight.

Health Insurance

Earlier, we briefly mentioned that "health insurance" and life insurance" should really be called *sickness insurance* and *death insurance* respectively. Or maybe call them both body insurance.

When we buy insurance for our home we get home owners insurance, we don't buy my-house-won't-burn-insurance as is indicated in the terms "health" and "life" insurance. *Health* and *life* do sound better than sickness or the more morbid sounding death insurance. But that is really what those insurances are, they are *sickness/accident* and *death* insurance, because generally, those are the circumstances that they are actually used for.

But "health" insurance is a peculiar thing. We have such insurance because we want to be protected when we get sick, but the insurance is not used to protect our health, it is intended to protect our finances, and that is a point that no one seems to realize about insurance.

Just like buying homeowners insurance will pay for a new roof when severe winds tear the roofing right off your home, health insurance will pay your hospital bill when you get sick–most of the time. But we do something peculiar with our health insurance that we don't do with our homeowner's insurance–we test it, *constantly*!

If you were to start your house on fire and call the fire department, then you would be jailed for arson and your homeowner's insurance company would likely cancel your policy and refuse to pay for the fire damages. But when it comes to health insurance that is exactly what we do, we test it. And if the legal penalty was that same for self-inflicted bodily sabotage as it is for arson, most of us would be in prison.

Your insurance is not there to make you well or keep you well; it's there to pay some of the medical bills that you might incur in the event of a major health emergency. It is a rare person who is careless when it comes to deliberately damaging their home and then expects the insurance to cover the damages. We all know that if we abuse our homeowner's insurance by repeatedly having wild parties that cause damage to our home, then eventually our homeowner's policy will be cancelled. But when it comes to our health insurance, we foolishly expect the insurance companies to pay again and again for every small expense that we caused with our careless attitude towards our bodies. The insurance companies would not mind paying all of our small medical expenses if we didn't abuse the policies as much as we typically do.

When we choose to develop eating habits that lead to being fat, then there are many medical expenses that arise, and we put the insurance companies on the hook for our horrible health-habits. This would be like smashing out couple of windows once a week or ripping off a few shingles and then getting the repairs done and submitting the bill to the insurance company. And if we are really obese, then it is closer in comparison to burning our house to the ground, repeatedly, and expecting the insurance companies to pay for it each time it is rebuilt.

To make matters worse, the government is trying to force insurance businesses to keep us insured even with our very bad health habits. If the insurance companies were forced by law to keep our homes insured, then everyone could repeatedly burn their home to the ground and everyone's homeowner's insurance rates would go up from hundreds of dollars per year to tens or hundreds of thousands of dollars per year, thus making the innocent pay for the actions of the guilty.

Regarding health insurance, the full costs surrounding a heart attack will cost more than the average home does. Let's take a look at a short list of health problems that can be caused or worsened by being too fat.

Arthritis

If we abuse our joints, we slowly wear down our cartilage between the joints causing us pain. This sometimes happens when we are too extreme in our workouts or in sports. Our joints need to be able to rebuild, but if we damage the cartilage too often, it doesn't have a chance to rebuild. If it can't ever rebuild we will destroy it beyond repair. This happens to athletes and sometimes in those who have jobs that required too much pressure too often on critical joints.

We also cause the same problem when we are over fat-weight. When we have more fat on our body than we should, then every time we stand up, all of our joints bear the extra pressure caused by the weight of our extra fat. The most dominant area where we hear people have problems with is at the knee. These problems are common mostly below and including the hips, knees, and ankles, but also your back.

In the long term, when we are in our golden years we will find those years not to be quite as golden as we might have imagined them to be, instead we end up with imperfect and painful years filled with joints that are ready to crumble far too early in life. Wearing away the cartilage that protects our bones due to unneeded stress from carrying the extra fat-weight often results in extreme joint pain and stiffness.

Back Problems

Depending upon the amount of excess fat we have and specifically where that excess fat is located, determines the amount and types of stresses on our backs. When we are over fat-weight we tend to position ourselves differently. And even though we might not realize that this is occurring, it will still cause unwanted wear and pain.

Even our mattresses suffer when we are over fat-weight. When we sleep on a mattress, the mattress will deform more if we are heavier and the excess mattress deformation can also put our body in a position that causes much unwanted back discomfort. We can buy a mattress designed for heavier people, but doing so is only a bandage on a wound that still has a thorn in it. To stop the bleeding, the thorn needs to be removed first, and only then can true healing begin.

Many of us suffer a great deal of back-discomfort due to our excess fat-weight, and the only true way to remedy that problem is to rid ourselves of the excess fat. Then over time, it is very likely that many of our pains will subside after our fat subsides.

Bones and Joints

In the arthritis section we mostly were referring to arthritis caused by too much pressure on our lower joints. But all of our bones and joints can be harmed by being over fat-weight. The stress is there 24 hours a day, 7 days a week, never resting always pressuring our joints and bones, but that is not the worst part.

The extra padding on the body does offer slightly more protection when we fall, but the excess weight increases the impact and the susceptibility of fracturing a bone. The worst part is that, if that broken bone is lower on the body, then the extra weight can inhibit healing, causing us to have sit, making us unable to get *any* exercise at all for a much longer time.

Cancers

The over fat-weight epidemic is relatively new to our modern medical world, and most of those studying this are still trying to figure out if there is a correlation with our health in relation to our weight. There are several types of cancer that have an increased susceptibility and are beginning to be associated with being over fat-weight. For women, these can include cancer of the breast, uterus, colon, and gall bladder. Over fat-weight men have a higher risk of colon and prostate cancer. But we can expect this list to grow as we grow our waistlines and as each new study comes out and is analyzed properly as they release more of the obvious correlations of excess fat and health problems.

Coronary Artery Disease

With increased fat-weight there is a higher risk of coronary artery disease. Coronary artery disease can be caused by the buildup of fat deposits or plaques in your arteries that lead to your heart. Eventually, these fat deposits narrow your heart's arteries, causing less blood flow to your heart. Decreased blood flow is bad because lower blood flow can cause chest pain. If your arteries get blocked completely you will have a heart attack.

Any restricted blood flow is going to inhibit your fat loss efforts. Eating right and getting safe amounts of exercises that are safe for each our personal condition is our best approach. The sooner we properly address the problem, then the sooner and faster we can get back to a healthy weight and a healthy body.

Type-Two Diabetes

Our over-fatness is a leading cause of type-two diabetes which used to be called adult-onset or noninsulin-dependent diabetes. Excess body fat causes the body to resist insulin. Insulin is the hormone that helps move sugar or glucose from our blood to individual cells. If the body is resistant to insulin, then our muscle cells can't get the glucose/sugar they need for energy, and then we tend to store that energy as fat all that much easier.

Gallstones

Gallstones are also statistically more common in people who are over fat-weight. But it's unclear how being over fat-weight results in gallstones. The reality likely is that it has to do specifically with the types of foods we eat and the quantity of them that we eat. But it could also have to do with chemical changes in our bodies that accompany being fat, possibly by not allowing the stones to dissipate or dissolve quickly enough to a point where excess fat and minerals build-up causing the stones to occur.

High Blood Pressure

When we have excess fat-weight we tend to retain sodium, then in order to dilute the sodium, we retain more water. This can increase our blood volume causing the pressure in our arteries to increase. This extra pressure causes the heart to have work harder. Excess fat-weight is also responsible for increases in heart rate due to the reduced flow through blood vessels to transport blood freely, which can also increase blood pressure and lead to hemorrhagic-stroke, the bursting of blood vessels in the brain.

When our blood pressure is high, our lives are at risk. *Some* high blood pressure is attributed to our eating habits directly, rather than our fat-weight being the cause, because even if we are thin, we can still have high blood pressure. But being over fat-weight contributes to our blood pressure issues, and if we don't want to pay the price with our quality of life, then the sooner we change our eating habits and lose the fat-weight, the sooner we can reduce all of the risks to our lives that are associated with our excess fat-weight.

Indigestion & Acid Reflux

Depending upon who you talk to, indigestion and acid reflux may be the same or slightly different. Nonetheless, they are almost always from excess eating or from bad eating habits in general–even if you are otherwise eating healthy. Eating too many and too much fatty items too quickly or too often, slows digestion causing the stomach to have hold food material that is difficult to digest for too long of a period. Some of this has to do with chewing our food well, as discussed in a previous chapter. When we chew well and eat reasonably well, then the food we consume digests quickly and properly, thus giving us the best yield for our food consumption with little or no discomfort.

The foods we eat should be moving along the digestive system quickly. But when the food fails to break down and is stuck in the stomach, then the stomach will produce more acid than would otherwise be needed, and it has the annoying habit of wanting to return the way it came in, especially when we lay down. Chew slowly, enjoy the flavor, and chew well, it helps digestion a lot! Eat less and live longer. Cut back on all caffeine including coffee, energy drinks, and soda along with sweet snacks and it is likely that you will lose, both, fat-weight and have reduced incidences of indigestion and/or acid reflux.

Also, as mentioned in an earlier part of this book, not eating right before bed can also help reduce or eliminate acid-reflux and indigestion when we lay down to sleep. Signs such as acid-reflux are like the warning lights on the dashboard of our vehicles which will be discussed in a following chapter.

Drinking far too much water can dilute the stomach's acidity too much and can also cause indigestion issues, and dumping coffee or other high caffeine products on top of that can make it worse. Healthy eating habits are all about proper balance.

Kidney Disease

Kidney disease can be made worse through bad eating habits and is made even worse when we are over fat-weight. Our kidneys are filters and when the filtering process is restricted in any way, it has a horrific effect on our health. Our blood is purified by our kidneys and when the blood cannot be properly cleaned, then the toxins that our bodies produce build up to dangerous quantities in our blood and will make us very sick.

When we overeat, or eat lots of low nutrient foods, it puts extra wear and tear on our organs, including on our kidneys. Our bodies have the most amazing ability to heal themselves when allowed enough time between eating to do so. But when we relentlessly infuse our bodies with excess food, the filtration mechanism never gets a reprieve.

The kidneys' filtration process never stops, and it is a matter of how much filtration is occurring. When the filtration process must filter too much contamination for too long and too often, then it is detrimental to our health, ultimately leading to many ill effects on the body.

Liver Disease

Damage to the liver through bad consumption habits takes a heavy toll on our entire system. When the liver is inhibited due to being diseased, then our digestion is affected and the nutrients that it creates or converts are also inhibited, causing our health to suffer greatly.

All of our organs are important, but the liver is an organ that we cannot live without and it is best to take good care of it by adopting reasonable eating and drinking habits. The contaminations taken from the blood and the nutrients infused into the blood by our organs are what keep us alive and healthy. Taking good care of these critical organs is much like taking good care of your car's engine, because without it running properly you're not going anywhere with it.

Pancreas Disease

When the pancreas is diseased, it negatively affects the chemistry needed for proper fat-weight loss and proper digestion. A diseased pancreas also inhibits the fat storage hormones and the very important insulin that regulates our blood sugar/glucose. Without a proper balance of these critical chemicals and hormones, our energy levels can be severely and negatively affected. If the blood sugar is not proper, we can feel groggy and have a foggy mind and can even go into insulin shock, causing all sorts of other problems, such as falling and hurting yourself from the fall when going into insulin shock.

Sleep Apnea

Sleep apnea is a problem that causes us to briefly stop breathing during sleep causing low oxygen levels which leads to drowsiness during the day and is, in general, not good for your body. Sleep apnea can also cause heart failure. Most of us who live with sleep apnea are overweight. The further over fat-weight we are then the more disruptive sleep apnea will typically be to us.

Besides the fact that it is generally bad for the body to have low blood oxygen, sleep apnea also tends to wake us and disturbs our sleep throughout the night making us groggy the next day, which only makes matters worse. It also could potentially cause your death due to suffocation.

Stroke

The building up of plaque in your arteries that feed the brain can eventually lead to a stroke if some other side effect of excess fat doesn't get to us first. When an artery leading to your brain becomes too narrow, then blood clots can form in the restricted area of the artery thus interrupting blood flow to the brain, ultimately resulting in an ischemic stroke. Being over fat-weight increases your chances of a stroke even in the absence of high blood pressure.

If you have ever known anyone who had a stroke, you are probably well aware of how devastating strokes can be. Strokes vary from little or no long-term ill effects all the way to severe paralysis of parts of the body, and even death.

The list of ailments that can accompany being over fat-weight is long and seemingly never ending. Being too fat has its financial costs as we have discussed, but the biggest cost of all is to our well-being. When our quality of life suffers, then everything else in our life will suffer along with it. But with a little bit of care and some simple changes in our habits, we can change the direction of our health with little or no effort–just a simple permanent change of habit.

Chapter 14

The Living Body Machine

The living breathing human body is a truly amazing invention. Even the bodies of animals are truly amazing. But the human spirit is uniquely different and gives a much greater value to the human body. But sadly, our world of "science" has stolen away much of the value of the human body and all of its wonders with their god-less Darwinian nonsense.

If we call the body a machine, then some religious people might get offended and the anti-religious people might say "I told you so". But the body is a mechanism of a highly sophisticated magnitude, and the designs and workings within the body are nothing short of pure genius!

Because we tend to either be in the religious group, or in the anti-religion group, we overlook the many functions of the body and how they can be used for our good. There are many functions *designed* into our bodies that are indicators of trouble, but because we don't look at the body for what it is, we tend to miss out on many of the body's built in features. Some of this is further discussed in *The Science Of God Volume 4 - Day Six - Evolution versus Man - In Our Image.*

The Dashboard of Your Body

Our bodies have many indicators and warning signs that are there as signs of danger for us. But too often we are removing those warning bells and warning lights by disconnecting them via improperly prescribed pharmaceutical bandages and/or our dangerous big-is-beautiful attitudes. Covering our warnings signs with drugs is okay to do if we realize the actual problem exists and address it and then deal with it and eventually eliminate those "medications".

If we have indigestion, then in probably more than ninety-nine cases out of one-hundred we have the power to stop the problem by changing when we eat, how much we eat, how often we eat, and what we eat, which includes all drinks.

The carry-over problems from something like acid reflux over long periods of time can have very negative over-all effects on our health.

Besides improper prescribing of medications, our ignorance is perhaps the largest contributor to our health and fat problems. The real problem with this comes due to our affinity for blaming *aging* for problems that are actually caused by *habits.*

There are many older people who have taken good care of themselves and at the age of eighty or even ninety or more they have few pains. They walk with a spring in their step and most of their good health has to do with their activity, eating, and attitude habits.

When we choose to blame things like acid reflux or any other fat related disease on aging, then we cheat ourselves out of being able to resolve those problems through a few basic changes in our habits. There are very few ailments that truly pertain to aging, most problems we have are related to our habits, including our fat-weight and all of the ill effects that excessive fat causes.

Women Are Different Than Men, Period

Despite what the world tries to tell us, women are different than men. Menstruation is often problematic for women when trying to lose weight. Since real fat-weight loss is based on energy spent, it takes time to lose weight. And unless you are working-out eight hours a day, it takes a several days to use enough calories to equal one pound of fat loss. This in itself is not the problem.

The problem with the female menstruation cycle occurs when fat actually has been lost, but due to the female cycle the female body tries to balance things to meet its needs caused by the cycle. Then often the result is the dreaded bloating and/or water retention. A one-hundred-fifteen-pound woman can easily retain a several pounds of temporary weight if she is experiencing bloating. But even this is not a problem in itself.

The problem is that when a pound or two of fat has been removed from the body and then due to the female menstruation cycle, the body retains water and waste, thus hiding the fact that the fat is actually gone. But even this is not the biggest problem; the real problem comes in when it discourages someone from continuing down the proper weight-loss path.

It is discouraging for a woman when she works hard for a couple of weeks and feels like she might actually be making visible progress, only to have the hard-earned progress disappear overnight due to water retention and bloating. This is why it is so important to log your efforts and to be honest about every single calorie you take in, and even more importantly to use DreamThin Averaging when recording your weight as explained in an earlier chapter.

Don't ever give up just because your weight went up several pounds overnight. If numbers are accurately recorded and you persist in your exercise and good eating habits, then when the bloating and water retention subside, you will see a new even lower fat-weight.

Be honest and trust your body, because your body with all of its wonderful indicators cannot tell a lie. Keep recording those numbers accurately and then after your body normalizes after the water retention and bloating are done, your weight will come right back down, and if you have been dedicated in your efforts and recording, then your fat-weight should be down lower than it was before the bloating began. Your scale will reward you with proper lower numbers!

It is important for men to understand how irritating this problem can be for women. It is a very frustrating and, often, uncomfortable situation. A good man will encourage and support their female counterpart, provided she is not unfairly and viscously verbally attacking him during those unfortunate mood swings. Women pay a heavy price in menstruation for being the gorgeous creations that they are. And all men should respect that!

Heat Up During Storage or Burning

As the body undergoes the various mechanical and chemical functions of fat-weight loss, you might notice some signs that something is happening. When the body is trying to use calories, one of the results is the production of heat even when at rest.

As the exchange of energy is occurring, it causes parts of the body to heat up. Depending upon how active you were during the day, your body is going to use energy and nutrients to repair the muscles; otherwise it will store that energy as fat. These processes can cause restlessness, itching, heating up, and sometimes even a bit of muscle pain.

We typically associate heating up with having consumed fast metabolizing substances such as sugar from drinking soda or eating sweets before bed. But regardless of what you eat, typically the body will heat up somewhat as it tries to burn that energy. Some of what cannot be burned through the heating process is likely to be stored as fat.

If on the other hand we are short calories and are ready for a night of dreaming ourselves thin, then we might also notice some heating up as the body begins to draw energy from our fat stores to use it to help rebuild muscle and sustain life. This too can be accompanied by itching or restlessness. When our muscles get hot, we tend to move around a lot at night in attempt to keep cool. Much of this occurs with the lower parts of the body because that is where our most powerful and largest muscles masses are that use most of our energy.

The body machine has these amazing indicators that we all need to become familiar with and learn to read. For every action we take with our eating and activity, there will be a reaction from the body. When we eat too much for our activity level to maintain a lower weight, then the body tells us this by our clothing getting tighter or maybe through indigestion etc. These sorts of indicators are not indicators of age or family DNA; rather they are indicators of our own bad habits.

Chapter 15

Details Everyone Should Agree On

There are a few details regarding fat-weight loss that everyone should agree on. The first and most important point to understand is that body fat will always and only be consumed or burned by the body when the calories being absorbed are less than the calories being used. This is simply a scientific and logical fact that applies to every human who ever was, is now, or will be.

The second is that there is no such thing as a "genetic predisposition to being fat", and being fat does not genetically run in anyone's family, but eating habits and personal honesty do tend to run in every family.

And last, fat and muscle weigh approximately the same. If you doubt this you can do a little experiment of your own and take two cups of tightly packed ground beef and two cups of butter and two cups of water and weigh each of them on an accurate kitchen scale. You will find them to be very much the same to a point of indifference–For all practical purposes, fat and muscle weigh the same per identical volume/size.

Health Vs Fat Weight Loss

In our blindly health conscious society, we often confuse health with fat-weight loss for the obvious reasons that it is unhealthy to be over fat-weight. But for fat-weight reduction purposes, we must to disconnect these two ideas.

For instance, bagels are not "healthy", they are food. If you butter it and sprinkle sugar on it, it has the same basic ingredients as a cookie does. Let's not fool ourselves into believing some things are healthy and others are not. Bread is the same; if you toast it, butter it, and sprinkle cinnamon sugar on bread you have just made a basic cookie. Eat a chocolate chip muffin with icing on it and you have cake.

Terms like "muffin", "bagel", or "whole wheat bread" are simply terms for the same basic thing with some rearranging of ingredients. When we add sugar and fat, then they are basically cookies or cake.

Nearly all baked goods consist of flour, eggs, fat, sugar, and flavoring to some degree. It is the arranging and mixing of the key ingredients that makes them each uniquely delicious, yet they all are about the same in general composition. So, don't allow yourself to be deceived. A large bagel may as well be a large donut because the calorie count is roughly the same. But it is worse with bagels and muffins and whole wheat breads because the serving sizes are often ridiculously huge due to the erred belief that they are "healthy", and all too often they contain several hundreds of calories. At least with a cookie we realize the fact that we are consuming the calories because of the negative stigma that cookies get. But this is unfair because many if not most bagels and muffins are served with added toppings, such as icing or butter, and they end up being far worse for our waistline than a simple cookie would have been.

Flour is flour regardless of what it is used to make and its calories do not change because we call it a "donut" versus a calling it a "bagel". The same is true of each ingredient. Consider all of the variations of pasta, they are all uniquely named, but all are made mostly of flour and formed into different shapes.

The health-versus-fat confusion goes far beyond what we choose to eat and lie to ourselves about regarding our food. Health and fat-weight are certainly connected, but are not necessarily the same. And the food supply chain takes advantage of our lack of knowledge about healthy products versus products aimed at our fat weight.

An important part of dreaming ourselves thin is to get a solid mental grasp on the *health* versus *fat-weight-loss* issue. When foods are promoted as "low-fat" we flock to those foods like flies to sugar. But reducing consumption of fat has little to do with fat-weight loss. We don't get fat from fat, we get fat from eating too much of ***anything***, but it is easier for us to get fat from consuming too much of the high-calorie-density foods.

These misunderstood sales points for the foods we buy and consume have more to do with *health* than with *fat-weight* loss. Most of the manufactured foods that are promoted as "healthy" because they are low-fat were originally targeted that way for the purposes of reducing cholesterol, and thus supposedly reducing clogged arteries that could induce a heart attack. But "low-fat" has mysteriously become the theme song of the weight-loss industry.

Our *health* versus our *fat-weight* has many points to be considered, but knowing that there is a difference is the key to unlocking the doors leading to what is a health concern versus what is a fat-weight concern.

Fat Thin People

Most of us have heard the term "fat-thin" people, but we might not have grasped its real meaning. We can calculate our personal perfect weight based upon the charts we find, but these charts cannot adequately gauge our own personal muscle mass.

Two adult bodies of the same gender, height, and age will have a skeletal structure that weighs about the same. While it is true that some people are "big boned", those differences are typically minimal regarding our total weight. Then we have our internal organs, and again those organs are fairly close in weight from person to person. But where we differ as people is in our habits, and those habits determine our muscle mass and the amount of fat we have.

Two people of the same personal perfect weight can look very different, because if one has lots of muscle mass they might have very little fat and look very fit, where another person of the same age, size, gender, and weight can have low muscle mass but have a high percentage of fat on their body and will tend to look a bit more saggy. It's when our muscle mass is too low that we can be a "fat-thin" person.

One way to solve this problem is to make sure you eat foods that will best contribute to increasing your muscle mass, but the real solution is for you to make sure that you use those muscles in such a way that they increase in size. As this occurs, the energy in your excess body fat will typically be consumed during the muscle-building process, thus allowing you to stay at a healthy weight while increasing the muscle as you lose the fat at the same time.

When we have too much fat on our body, our systems must work harder no matter how much we weigh. So if we have low muscle mass, but have too much fat and yet are at a personal perfect weight, then it is very possible that we can suffer from the same health issues that other people who are over fat-weight and over their perfect weight suffer from.

This is why the scale is thought to not be important to some people, but it is important and we should use it to help us understand our own body. Your personal perfect weight is something that should be determined with much understanding and possibly with the help of a nutritionist, trainer, or physician.

Getting our body fat down to a personal good general level will make us healthier, giving us a clearer view of what is hidden under all of our fat. If your muscle mass ranges between low to extremely low, then you considering thinking about doing exercises to build those muscles is probably a good idea. This is not referring to excessive professional body-building here, but rather getting the body to a healthy state so that it can burn calories more quickly, and also have the strength to do the same tasks most other people can do.

Your System, Less In, Less Out

You will notice changes in your system as you adjust your eating habits. Probably a more prominent change will be your restroom "regularity". The less we eat, then the less we need to visit the restroom. This is normal. Do not get this confused with constipation. If you don't eat much, you likely won't poop as often, this is not constipation. In fact, while not recommended, if a person took in only the exact calories their body needed, and those calories where in the form of sugars, then the need to use the restroom would be almost nonexistent. But this would not be healthy for anyone's body. It is important that our systems pass foods through on a somewhat regular basis as a sort of God-given purifying mechanism to keep our bodies healthy.

When going without food while doing longer-term fasting, we typically notice that when we eventually eat, we experience intestinal gas problems. There are several reasons for this, but the main reason is that when the system is very empty, the food we eat is able to travel through our system faster than normal because it's empty. This causes undigested food to prematurely get into areas where the digestion is handled differently. When the system is empty and then suddenly filled with food, the food can be distributed all throughout the digestive system quickly allowing more gassing in a shorter period of time. When gassing of the intestinal contents is minimal, then the body absorbs some of it or the aspects that cause the gas. But if too much is produced too quickly, then it tends to demand its way out.

This can occur if you don't eat for several days and then you suddenly eat a lot. Doing so can also cause you to have to suddenly rush to the restroom in utter urgency. It is not recommended to suddenly eat a lot after a longer fast, so when eating after a fast, starting modestly can be of some help and is wise to consider doing in that case. There are no recommendations for a total no-food fast, but when we fast for God, we are told to take the money or food saved from the sacrifice of fasting and give it to someone in need while we offer thanks to God.

People often misunderstand fasting or do it wrong. For dieting purposes when done wrong it can be damaging to your health. So, understanding what "fasting" is can help you to understand your body and what will occur when you fast. For some people, a "fast" is complete absence of eating any food for their chosen time-frame. For others fasting is simply depriving one's self of something such as chocolate. You can find opinions on the fasting subject ranging from one extreme to the other. But regardless of whether or not you choose to fast, or just cut back a bit, don't confuse your past restroom regularity with your current fasting's reduced restroom visits, where you think it is constipation. It probably is not.

Less in, less out is the general rule. And being aware of this can help you gauge if your body is functioning as expected or if you have other issues to deal with.

Getting It to Pass Through Your System

It is good to have our digestive system function in such a way that we are passing the used food through it with reasonable regularity. This helps us keep the toxin levels in the body low, which assists in keeping us healthy. But when we eat less, we go less, and this sometimes causes the used food matter to stay in the digestive system too long. Sometimes we might feel a bit off when this occurs, so eating fruits is usually helpful, or any other particular food that tends to cause the need for you to visit the restroom.

When the body processes the foods that we consume, it exchanges fresh nutrients for used toxins that are produced by the functioning of the body. These toxins are either sweated out or they are excreted out when we visit the restroom. But when we are not reasonably regular, the toxins that are contained in our waste will sit within the digestive system and can be partially reabsorbed, making us feel ill or groggy. This is why "eating right" is important for all of us.

The right types of foods at the right times, helps to produce the bile that aids in digestion and it helps with the elimination of our body waste. We can eat whatever we want, but getting the proper nutritional needs from the foods that we do eat is very important to both our health and to our fat-weight loss efforts. If what you want to eat on a regular basis lacks the required nutrition that your body demands, then you can expect to have health issues in the long run.

How Long Will It Take to Lose this Fat-Weight?

When dreaming thin you can calculate the fat-weight loss completion date to within a few weeks accuracy provided that you are honest and accurate with *all* entries when recording calories used and calories consumed. The time it takes is really quite mathematical when you are very precise in your estimating and recording of calories. If you run a calorie deficit of only 100 calories per day then it will take 35 days to lose a pound of fat-weight. But if you increase that deficit to 400 calories by taking an hour-long daily jog, then you can lose a pound in just over eight days. Your pounds of fat-weight beyond your personal perfect weight can be multiplied by 3500 calories in a pound of fat, and that can be divided by your daily calorie deficit to estimate how many days it will take to lose your desired amount of fat-weight at that particular calorie deficit.

If someone is forty pounds over fat-weight, then they have stored 140,000 calories and that can be divided by their 400-calorie daily deficit, resulting in approximately 350 days to lose the 40 pounds. Sure, we want to do it faster, but most of us have been trying to unsuccessfully deal with the problem for decades. But if we stay true to our goal for only a single year, we can have our cake and eat it too, literally! And we can do so without being fat.

Your Equilibrium

Depending upon your eating habits, you may be at what DreamThin refers to as "equilibrium", which is where you have not been gaining anymore weight, but you might be overweight. The theory being, that your present activity level plus your present fat content level balances with your current eating habits.

But don't be fooled by thinking you are at equilibrium, because as was discussed earlier in this book, we generally put weight on at only a few pounds per year and we barely notice that it's occurring. For fully grown adults, when clothes get tight it is an indicator that it is now time to lose fat-weight. It is *not* an indicator to buy larger clothes.

Technical Tidbit

The concept of DreamThin is accuracy and constancy, but because we humans have an inclination to inaccurately estimate eating and activity, much to our fat loss disadvantage, some people choose to figure 4,000 calories per pound of body fat to compensate for their inaccuracy rather than the 3,500 actual calories that body fat is. Most errors and miscalculations of calories by vendors and consumers can be compensated by using the 4000 calorie per pound index. But when someone chooses to do this, their goal weight stays the same. However, as the personal perfect weight is approached, then re-evaluation of the current tone and build of your body must be done, and if you have any doubts about what is right then consult with a nutritionist-physician or trainer and your mirror and the wise opinion of wise friends, if you actually happen to have a few *wise* friends.

Scales are important indicators, but the truth is shown in a quality mirror that accurately reflects your new-improved self. Never use the scale for final analysis when you are at or near your perfect weight. If you find that you want your body to be toned then you might need to choose do certain exercises during losing the fat or after the fat is gone.

Ask Your Doctor before Making Changes in Life Habits

After you have read and fully understand the DreamThin concept, it is suggested that you seek your physician's approval before starting any fat-weight reduction efforts.

Your end goal is to be *properly* thin ***and healthy***; doing anything that might injure or harm you in anyway will be of no help to your getting fit. Some people have a very good assessment of their own body and what will be safe eating and exercise practices for themselves, but most of us don't asses ourselves properly, which can be safely inferred by the size of our waists. The last thing any of us want is to be injured and unable to take a simple walk or jog; or worse, to cause harm to any of our vital organs by failing to get proper daily nutrition. This is why most, if not all, weight-loss programs insist that we visit a physician and get good medical advice before we start. This is just good advice all around, especially if you have any uncertainties at all.

And it is best if you can find a physician that is specifically trained in nutrition, but they are somewhat rare.

Can I Really Lose Weight While I Sleep?

Can I really lose fat-weight while I sleep? Yes, this was discussed in an earlier chapter. The whole point of the term "DreamThin" is that we can lose weight during the hours at night when we sleep and dream. All we need to do is to make sure our digestive system has been mostly emptied and then begin eating fewer calories per day than we use per day, and also to make sure that the late evening or late-night snacking is very minimal or eliminated altogether. When we do this, it allows for a long enough period of time for the body to be forced to burn off fat at night, rather than storing the food we consume at night as fat.

If our calorie intake is very close to our calorie needs, then simply making this change can cause most people to begin to lose weight by doing nothing more than the simple change of ***not*** eating several hours before bed.

Chapter 16

Seeing Through the Lies

What's a better term for food extremists: food nazis or food police? Both are true, and under either name those people are annoying as hell. All food is good food, and it is only the quantity of the food that we eat that is helpful or harmful.

A Ridiculous Notion

Food alarmists will shame you for doing something as simple as cooking your veggies. But what they fail to understand is that when foods are prepared through any one of various methods of heating, then other very helpful nutrients can be created during that process, and those nutrients are just as beneficial as the nutrients when in an uncooked form.

Sensationalized stories are told for dramatic effect so that the media can make us stop and say "Wait... What was that?... You mean to say that cooked carrots are bad for your health?" This is a well-known practice in the news and publications industries. Being "shocking" in effort to grab our attention is a tactic that has been paying them well for centuries. But then *we* are left with the result of our response to it, which only serves to cause more of their nonsensical hype.

The Food Police

Food police is not really the best term for these annoying people, because police are good and attempt to stop us from doing stupid stuff. "Food nazi", on the other hand, is a more appropriate term because a nazi demands that you do things their way. Earlier in this book the subject of refrigeration was brought up and how it revolutionized the world. It is this refrigeration revolution that allows the foolish food nazi to flourish. They don't flourish because of refrigeration, but rather they flourish in spite of refrigeration.

The food nazis, might be your neighbor or a friend, or even a family member. They are typically not concerned about your fat-weight or concerned for what that can do to your health, rather they are concerned only with *their own view* of how *you* should live and what you should eat.

There are many factions of the food nazis. There are juicing-purist-nazis that insist that juicing is the salvation of all things. Then we have the never-cook-your-veggies-nazis, and the never-eat-fruit nazis, then there are the no-carbs-nazis, and let us not forget the no-dairy-nazis or the no-meat-nazis. But probably the most irritating are the you-must-become-a-vegetarian-nazis and they are challenged by the everyone-must-become-a-vegan-nazis. But the most dangerous are the eat-only-organic nazis. Oh, and let's not forget the no-poultry-nazis or the eggs-will-give-you-a-heart-attack-nazis and the butter-will-kill-you-nazis and the no-processed-food-nazis. Wait there's more, we have the you-can't-sell-soda-in-this-city-nazis and the you-can't-sell-large-sodas-nazis, and the list goes on and on and on and on and on... There is always some moron spouting off their foolish perspective trying to misguide our ways. Avoid the confusion and ignore these ignorant people.

Food is food and eating it with joy *in reasonable quantities* while making sure that you are getting enough of the required nutrients for your body to function efficiently is all that anyone really needs to know short of having some rare disease or allergy that certain foods can aggravate.

What the food nazis, who stand in accusation of each of our cuisines miss is that this is all new. Why does this matter? It matters because prior to about 1920, few people had refrigerators, and even if they would all have had them, the electrical infrastructure at that time, could not have handled the capacity of the extra power required. This means that foods were either very expensive to deal with or had a very short shelf-life. This in itself was not a problem. People simply went to the market and bought foods from the local grocer who bought them from the local farmer; and they did this more often than we need to do today.

Many people even had gardens in the backyard. Paradise, right? No so fast! Fresh food was not a problem for those who lived in rural areas and had room for a garden or access to fresh produce. But let's consider the problems this caused the millions of people clustered together in the big cities. Fresh food delivery to these areas was not an easy task. Only a little over a hundred years ago food was being brought in from local farms on horse and carriage into New York City! The people in the city likely paid more for their food and likely had produce that was not nearly as fresh as the rural communities did, and much of it may have been near to ready to spoil.

Spoiled foods are dangerous for people to eat and can cause sickness and even death. Prior to trucking and refrigeration, percentage-wise, many more people became ill from poor nutrition issues and food poisoning etc. than happens today.

It was a mission of the government and manufacturers to come up with solutions for a rapidly growing population who were becoming sicker as the population grew larger and more dense. This made vitamin-fortified products such as cereal very useful and helpful to us as a nation. As refrigeration came into play, we could now store veggies and many other foods for extended periods of time.

By the time refrigeration was finally affordable, preserved and packaged goods had already become commonplace in our lives. Initially this was not a problem. In fact, up until about 1970 this was extremely beneficial to the citizens of the United States and the entire globe. People's health was stabilized and they were not dying as often from malnutrition and its related problems, or from food poisoning in developed areas.

We miss this issue today because we focus on increasing instances of cancer, but we fail to realize that we are no longer dying from diseases of past times that occurred at ages far too young like was happening in days gone by.

What the food nazis need to understand is that if only one of their ancestors had died from starvation, malnutrition, or food poisoning they would not be here condemning the rest of us. And the relatively modern wonders of the food chain are likely what allowed them to survive.

Years ago many people suffered from lack of nutrients. Unless you could cost-effectively get abundant and proper fresh veggies etc. to your door, sufficient protein was hard to come by. This made meat a very efficient means to store and keep protein. Meat, cheese, and grain were all a very big deal in solving nutrition problems seen in areas where produce was difficult to effectively deliver year-round. Once the meat and dairy *industry* was born, refrigeration only added to its growth. In effort to keep this country strong, we wanted to make sure the citizens did not starve again, and this was dependent upon a stable ability to produce foods.

The people who started many of the major corporations that supply our foods today, started those companies before refrigeration was common, and they did a wonderful service for all of humanity in doing so. These people made great amounts of profit and they deserved great amounts of profit. We can even extend this over to restaurants like McDonalds and grocers like Wal-Mart.

So, where did the problem come in and when did some people turn into the food nazi brigade? During the late 1960s and the 1970s manufacturers wanted to make more money and began to have idle time and wanted to grow their businesses. The food chain was full, and the nation was healthy! This brought on many new convenience foods, luxury foods, comfort foods, and excess!

While we might want to condemn and accuse these major corporations who employ a great portion of the citizens of this country, we need to understand how they came to be. If they were suddenly wiped out of existence, then rampant starvation and malnutrition would occur inside of a single year. We need these companies. Not only do many people not know how to garden in our modern age, but, in general, as a population, we are too lazy to do so.

Once the supply pipeline was full and everyone had eaten their fill, the companies suddenly experienced the dreaded business growth-lull. If profits are high in percentage this is not a problem. But, when profit-margin parentages are low due to being built on a model of constant expansion/growth, companies that have a massive workforce must maintain buildings and equipment and keep selling product. At this point a lull in business becomes a serious financial liability for them. This causes these companies to realize that if they want to survive and not go broke they must lay off many people who will then no longer have jobs, they then had better find a way to sell more product. Enter the 1970's!

During the 1970's the country was flourishing. People where mostly healthy and had money from working at the food manufacturers, etc. and had spare time and spare cash. We were caught up on our work as a country and it was now time to celebrate. And celebrate we did!

As the manufacturers began to feel the unprofitable pinch of a full pipeline, they began to produce convenience foods in mass. This stepped up production of new and old items and it worked for about ten years. At that point, because our production and delivery methods were so efficient, the pipeline was once again filled full and even overflowing in only about ten years, but this time with convenience foods.

What happened next is that in the 1980's the manufacturers again now felt the painful profit-lull of a full food-chain pipeline. Once the delivery mechanism of fast-food chains and mega grocers had saturated the market with their many locations, they faced the same profit-lull fate as the food manufacturers did. Since their low profit-margin business models were based upon absolute continued growth, this presented a problem for them. It's easy to grow as a business when you can continue to build store after store where you don't really have to concern yourself with what is on the menu, or the selection of goods in the store. This unbridled growth led to our current-day problem of over-eating. What's the next step after full and absolute market penetration and complete saturation? Over-abundance!

When a market is full and fully saturated, then the only way to continue to grow is to sell more. And how do you sell more? Once the market is saturated and everyone is healthy and has eaten full, you need to sell them an upscale meal.

Enter the Big McWhopper! At two to three or more times the price and calories of a standard basic burger, this technique allowed food supply-chain companies to continue to see profit growth. This caused us to buy more and more at lower prices for more food. And buy we did. We did this all through the 1980's,

1990's and 2000's and we continue to do this into the 2010's, 2020's, and beyond.

For more than forty years we have been over-eating as a nation; and what once saved our lives is now taking our lives. This is nobody's fault in particular, and it is certainly not the food's fault. It simply happened and will continue to happen.

Enter the food nazis. The food nazis can blame the Wal-marts and McDonalds' of the world, but that will not solve this problem. Instead, we must take it upon ourselves to resist some of the wonderful robust selections they have to offer us. Such companies could increase their profit by raising their prices and reducing portion sizes, but then the food-price-nazis will scream "price gouging!"

It is us who decide that we are going to eat two of everything that they have to offer. It is ***our*** choices that cause the problem with our health. This health, cancer, and fat-weight problem that now plagues us is not the fault of the food producers. Most of us would be dead without them.

We complain about high prices, and then we get hypocritically angry at these companies for selling us two jumbo size items for the price of one. Either we want good prices or we don't. We must stop oscillating on these issues.

The cost to package a small item and deliver it to us is almost the same as the cost to package a large item and deliver it to us. This means that food suppliers can offer larger quantities for close to the same price just as we request. It is not their fault, *it's* ***our*** *fault.*

We want food, cheaper, sweeter, and saltier and they produce what we want. When they try to manufacture and sell alternate healthier choices we respond by ignoring it, not buying it, and letting it go bad on their shelves. Why, then, do the food nazis expect the food producers to offer what we refuse to buy?

In the Bible, when the people wandered in the desert for forty years, the Creator laid down instructions for them to only collect one day's needs of food for their household and to each eat only their share and remove any excess from the house that had not been eaten that day. If I recall correctly, those who took more than was instructed had their leftovers turn rancid and become worm-infested. There was a limit of how much they were supposed to eat each day! This is a lesson that we, today, do not want to hear, and we are going to demand less money for more food until we eat ourselves ***dead***!

Now, not only do we take more than a day's worth of food, but we eat more than a day's worth of food. If the Creator made the excess that they disobediently kept go bad in the cup, then do we imagine that any less will occur in our stomachs? Do these rules no longer apply? Gluttony is greatly frowned upon in the Bible. We are gluttons and we must admit it! We are like the Israelites demanding that Moses (the food companies) approve our bad habits and then we blame him (the food companies) when we get fat.

It is time for us to pull our heads out of the desert sand and assume responsibility for our own hands *and* mouth! The food nazis who shout and blame, blame, blame have no clue as to history or what is involved with delivering fresh quality produce into our hands. Not everyone lives in rural areas and not everyone can afford high-nutrient natural foods.

A good suggestion is, instead of complaining and blaming everyone, those who are screaming about what they think we should eat, should properly educate themselves and then offer their own money to their fellow man for proper foods. And in the unlikely event that they actually possess the knowledge, the food nazis should try to educate, instead of accusing and blaming the producers of the foods that allow us live the life of convenience and luxury that we and they all live and enjoy today.

The various food nazi groups are far more blind than they will ever imagine, nor do they understand the dynamics of food delivery and preparation in metropolitan areas. And they do not understand the complications that this country faced with regard to malnutrition and disease during its history.

Let's propose a challenge to the various food nazi groups who are more of *acting*, than of *action*: Start your own food company! And if you don't like the system, then ***you*** produce a menu of foods that are healthy and have a shelf-life so that they can be there for those who don't own a farm or land of their own on which to plant food to sustain life. And then try to have those foods last on the shelf so that your customers don't get food poisoning or otherwise sick from eating your offerings that are rotting on the shelf because they have not been properly preserved so that the customers don't decide to sue you for your incompetence. Harsh? Yes! But true.

We can have a blind and arrogant heavenly-paradise view of each man having his own garden and planting enough food for the year, but tell us, how exactly will you keep that produce fresh? And what will you do when you live north of Springfield, Illinois and it gets too cold to grow food for about six months out of the year? Will any food nazis give us their own land down south where we can grow our food year-round? Not likely.

The food suppliers are not going to complain when you buy more, nor do they have the time or the right to say "Hey, you're too fat mister, I refuse to serve you!" If they did restrict us and refuse to serve us because we are too fat, then the discrimination-nazis would sue them for discrimination.

Food manufacturers put ingredients in foods for a few reasons: To preserve them, to actually make them, and to enhance their flavor. And for this the food nazis accuse them of making the food "addictive". Falling prey to the blame-game keeps us fat and unhealthy and *will not* change the menus or our health.

It is up to *us* to drink only a twelve-ounce soda cup of with ice per visit instead of drinking a forty-ounce soda *without* ice per visit. Blaming our "addiction" to food on the food suppliers is only going to keep us fat and unhealthy and serve to make us fatter and unhealthier.

Continuing to grab that bag of chips when we walk out of the store is seen as a vote for chips by the chip manufacturer. Each bag of chips is a vote for chips, and if we stop voting for it they will stop electing to make it for us–problem solved!

Those who blame, will remain as they are, with some being stupid, some fat, and some others dead due to ignorance. Many of us eat enough per day for two or three and even four people. Take it upon yourself to save your own life, and as it was instructed to the people in the Bible: eat only *your* share for the day (See Exodus 16:18).

Ignore the many food nazi groups who seek to steal your joy by limiting *your* food choices to *their* distorted palate.

Their Agenda

Some of the food nazis are hired by organizations that have an interest in getting us to utilize their product through demonizing other competing products. But most food nazis are misguided people who have strong opinions and have little or no understanding of reality, of health, or of business.

The food nazis that are hired by companies are often hired by firms that promote the various dieting programs, and those programs will demonize any food that does not fit with their program, essentially frightening us into eating what they say and sometimes sell. This is not to say that these products are not of some use, but let us understand that some of the information that we get from these particular food nazis is agenda-based and is financially driven.

Dangers of Extremism

As for the armchair food nazis, we are all best to ignore their foolish insistence, and instead make sure that what we eat, we eat in modest and appropriate quantities. As we have witnessed over the years, many of these food nazi people ironically die at ages that are far too young while the rest of us live on.

The joy of food is a gift from God that we should all enjoy every day in modest portions so that we can continue to enjoy it every day for a very long life, giving thanks for it every time we eat.

Extremism almost always ends in failure, and often it ends in death. Don't become one of the food nazis! Enjoy your own life and allow others to enjoy their own lives as well. If you ever promote anything, then promote modest portions and getting enough of the required nutrients.

Do Not Make Food Out to Be Evil.

Do not make food out to be evil. Doing so will only cause your children and those who foolishly believe you, to rebel inside when they discover how tasty these treats are. Teaching others how to choose wisely and eat modestly is the key.

Prohibition usually fails in the long term, but proper knowledge and solid understanding never fail for those who practice it and seek Truth.

All Food is Good

All food is wonderful, and in the Bible God wanted us to feast. We were supposed to bring offerings to the priest and celebrate with friends, family, and the priest once in a while. The problem is that, the same way that you can use your car to drive to work or drive off a cliff, you can use food to share Joy once in a while and maintain a healthy DreamThin figure, or you can drive off the proverbial fat-cliff by eating too much until your body can no longer handle the stress and you get cancer, diabetes, high blood pressure, fat, and heart conditions, etc.

It's our choice for Joy or for death. Too much of a good thing is usually bad. Think about it... Anything we overindulge ourselves in results in self-destruction: alcohol, sex, spending money, and even work. We should take only our own daily allowance of whatever we do.

When did we lose the lesson of moderation taught to us in the Bible that has worked for thousands of years for billions of people? All food is a wonderful gift and should be treated as the privilege that it is, then we will automatically DreamThin when following the basic rule of ***moderation***.

Never blame food for *your* fat-weight problems if you ever want to dream yourself thin. Only personal responsibility can solve our problems regarding our fat-weight. When we listen to the food nazis and we blame the food or the food makers, we then ignore the real problem and keep on eating. Manufacturers and retailers might change our mind regarding what foods we eat, but generally not the quantity that we eat. Any one of us is capable of losing fat-weight when we face the truths regarding the foods that we eat and we eat only that which the body ***needs***.

Chapter 17

Sharing Your Experience

Some of the food nazis are people who have over-indulged in their favorite foods and overcome their own fat-weight problems using a certain diet. They then want to share this with others who have the same problem, but insist that we do it their way.

It is important that we share our successes with others because it gives them hope that they too can get fit and be the proper personal weight and be all around healthier. But if we turn them off and become food or exercise nazis, it is very discouraging to them.

Learn the required knowledge and understand it all properly before you share it. It is okay to share what you did, but don't dictate what others must do. It is only when you truly *understand* that you are then able to properly help others with sound advice.

Social Problems

In a world that equates thinness with beauty, intelligence, and success, fat adults will often experience unfair psychological stress, lower income, and discrimination. It's sad to say, but it's true. It is in the best interest of most businesses to not hire over fat-weight people. While fat people are just as talented as thin and fit people, being fat slows productivity and is very expensive for companies who offer insurance to their employees.

Being fat is also very humiliating, and in our modern day of social media and the cruelty that goes along with it, many people are emotionally destroyed indirectly by the general sentiment found on social media.

But the problem gets worse, because now if you are fat you will either feel horrible because of what people say, or maybe you will embrace the foolish "big-is-beautiful" mantra that has been born out of social media that is basically telling you that it is good or cool to be fat. Choose to be fat if you like, but don't imagine that there are no social, financial, and medical costs to be paid for that choice. And never ask the rest of the community to pay for your own bad eating habits.

Fear of Your Past

Our past should be one of the most cherished resources we have. It might sometimes be painful, but it is nonetheless valuable. Never fear your past, because it is your road map of what to avoid in your future. Your past can be used to help yourself, and others, avoid the unpleasantries of life. It is when we use our past to avoid those past mistakes in our future that gives it such tremendous value for our future. The book *Hot Water - Your Perceived Identity - The Life Repair Manual* discusses this in more detail.

Using Your Past

When we use the road map of our past, we need not dwell on it and cause ourselves to frustrate our efforts by constantly recalling our errors and troubles. It is to be used as our index.

And if our past was not particularly wise in direction, then we must use it to redirect our future to a wise outcome. So, let us not forget that our past most certainly also has good things in it, proving that we can also use those good things to gauge where we want to be in the future.

Master Your Past

We have mastered our past when we use it for only good and to avoid the potholes of life. It is with the wisdom learned from our past mistakes that we actually become wise.

Sadly, there are too many of us that hide ourselves in the humiliation of our past. This problem is becoming worse with the unrelenting and lasting memory of "social media".

Wisdom tells us to do our best and to not do stupid things, and it tells us even more so, don't record yourself doing or saying stupid things for the world to see on social media.

Mastering our past is the act of learning from our past mistakes and becoming wise from that learning, thus enabling us to understand the consequences of any future actions we might take, especially our eating actions.

In a Perfect World

Yes, in a perfect world we would all help each other and watch out for each other. But, sadly, we are a self-serving bunch of beings that are all out for ourselves foraging for food. So, the "next big kill" as human evolution supporters would put it, is when our steering wheel spins us into the nearest drive through, though, I don't agree that we evolved to seek out such foods.

To forage and go for the kill is more of a "we evolved" perspective. Since we were actually designed by the Creator to discover and know the Creator, it is unlikely that we were designed to seek out the next big kill. But in our attempt to want more, or seek more, via the knowledge of good and evil, Eve, and then Adam, and finally all of humanity placed ourselves in a shortage mentality. We never think we are good enough, and this mental functionality filters through and trickles down throughout all of our actions and in everything in our lives. We cannot avoid this unless we individually choose to do so. If we do it in one area of life, then we likely do it to some extent in all other areas of our life. This means that if we believe that we are not good enough or not smart enough, then there is a high likelihood that we feel as if we do not have enough in other areas of life. The result of this will be to attempt to fulfill the shortage or void by doing something such as eating more. And some foods, due to the chemistry involved, certainly cause us to not feel sated. Generally, we don't think about this in these terms, but it is true nonetheless.

So, the part in the Bible where they are told to only take their day's portion is indicative of our design. Which is to say, to eat our share, and eating only our share is a part of our biological design. It is abusing our design that makes us fat. If, in fact, we were designed to forage for food and eat what we could until the next big kill, then we would be able to eat and not have it adversely affect us. But this does not happen, which clearly tells us that this fat, that too many of us now wear on our waistlines, was designed and intended for balance, something that we abuse to great extents.

Be a Part of the Solution

We all have the choice to be a part of the solution, or to be a part of the problem. Most of this comes through planting seeds of understanding in the hearts and minds of our fellow man. We can be a part of the big genetic lie that "We are born with some sort of fat-gene", or we can thwart that lie and defy it and show those around us that it is not true. We can show them the truth by using the fundamental science of–energy used verses energy consumed. Then we can be their example to light their way to truth.

Chapter 18

Our Desires

Oh, we humans have desires alright, and many of them can be bad for us when abused. When we tame our desires or shift the focus of those desires, then we can transform our own personal world of hurt to a world of wonder! Desire is a true gift that we have been Created with, but when we abuse our desire we abuse that gift.

One of the biggest problems that we face with our desires is that we often adopt other peoples' desires as our own because we want to be like them. This is not necessarily a bad thing, but we really should develop our own desires.

We also have an issue with regard to our desire as to how we should look when we lose our fat-weight. Most people have reasonably realistic view of what they want to see in the mirror when their own goal is finally accomplished.

Can Someone Be Too Thin?

One dangerous area of our weight-loss desires is the mental and emotional distortion we sometimes have regarding how thin we should be, or how we mentally visualize ourselves in the mirror.

Some people are so traumatized by having been fat that they always see themselves as too fat no matter how thin they become. This affects them to a point where they become anorexic. Some of this is a call for attention, but sometimes it is a true mental distortion. These situations are not helped by the various forms of media that most young women are exposed to.

Every person is beautiful just as they were Created. The opinions of the world are irrelevant regarding our own self and our self-worth. We must take care of our self-image and our self-worth, and when we have those two squarely in place then it is far easier to for us to deal with issues surrounding our fat-weight.

The excessively skinny look of a true anorexic is very unappealing and is easily solved by eating right and eating enough. When people eat too little for too long, it causes the body to consume itself including our muscle mass. When we allow our muscle mass to be consumed, we look sickly and become weaker, unattractive, and unable to do many tasks we previously were readily able to do.

What I want anorexic women to know is that true beauty has nothing to do with how thick or thin we are. To truly love yourself, you also have to take proper care of yourself. People who care for and love themselves are generally easier to love. When we hate ourselves, or our bodies, then we tend to push others away from us causing us to feel unwanted and unloved all the more, but it is our own fault when we do this and it is very easy to correct.

Yes, we can be too thin and it is bad for the mind, the body, our health, and for our social interaction with everyone around us. When we adopt the ridiculous idea that there is no God and that we have evolved from primates, then we have no true value and are no better than the animals. But this is **not** true!

The only true value we have as humans is the fact that we have been Created and the fact that we are unique individuals that are Created in the image of the Creator. Our worth is beyond all money or status and has no value that can be measured when we simply follow God and Truth. (See *Hot Water - Your Perceived Identity - The Life Repair Manual)*

People Tell You to Eat More, But...

If you read enough weight-loss and exercise articles, you are bound to come across those articles that will tell you to eat more calories. This is true and it can work with proper foods and proper understanding, but you must fully understand what you are doing or you will end up only gaining even more fat-weight.

When we're told to increase our calories and eat as much as we want, then there are certain important technical points that accompany doing so. Typically, that advice comes along with much exercise, and a food selection heavy in veggies and certain carbs.

If you are going to eat more, then you must eat *properly* as they instruct, which is very important. If you decide that you are going to eat a three or a four thousand calorie daily diet you must not eat certain kinds of food. Some foods increase the body's metabolism and this appears to be true by most studies regarding such diets. But when we eat the food for this sort of diet, but are also eating foods that are high in sugar and fat for instance, then this extra energy is often held in the body and is absorbed and stored as fat.

*Understand **all*** of the details of any diet and how those details affect your body before attempting to adhere to the diet. If we don't fully understand the diet that we choose, then small inadvertent discrepancies will actually cause us to gain weight rather than lose weight.

Consider the issues that can arise with the "Atkins" or "keto" diet. The point of these diets is to reduce carbohydrate intake to a very low level which will put the body into a state of ketosis. When the body is in ketosis it burns fat rather than storing the energy as body fat. This diet works well for many people, but fails miserably for many others.

Why does it work for some and not for others? It's because some people don't do details well and they do not understand the stringent nature of the diet. You are allowed very few grams of ***any*** carbohydrates with this type of diet. If you violate that basic rule, then you will end up gaining weight and sometimes that fat-weight will come on with a vengeance. Depending upon your size and gender, the amount of grams of carbohydrates allowed in a day typically ranges from about only thirty to sixty grams. A single bagel has about seventy, so if you want a ketosis diet to work properly, you are limited to about a half of a bagel per day. If you exceed that, *then the diet won't work.* So, if you have two bagels per day on that sort of diet, then you will likely gain weight quickly.

If you do the keto-type diet properly then you can eat as much meat and fat as you want. However, since most of the variety in food comes with carbohydrates, it makes these ketosis type diets very boring after a very short time.

Cut Soda and Diet Soda

Diet soda is perhaps the biggest contributor to weight gain, especially in females. Why would diet soda cause weight gain, you ask? It's because if you're like most of us, you have been sort of watching what you eat and likely have been somewhat conscious of how many calories you are consuming daily, but have probably been losing track at around the one-thousand calorie mark each day. So, you think "I'll drink diet soda instead to keep my calories down" but you eat more because you removed the soda calories, thus ending up having only replaced the soda calories with food calories, which is not a good idea.

Often when we are a little bit overweight and not gaining, but are counting calories and do not want to gain fat-weight, we decide to start drinking diet soda instead of regular soda. But then we covertly feel that we can eat more food each day because of the calorie reduction from switching from regular to diet soda. When we do this, it is very likely we will quickly start gaining fat-weight.

Sugar from the soda is typically processed quickly by the body and causes the body to heat up or causes us to have a sudden burst of energy. But when we replace regular soda with diet soda, we then end up replacing those soda calories with other carbohydrates or fat, which are far more likely to get stored as body fat energy.

The idea of diet soda is to not change anything in your eating habits provided you are consuming the proper amount of calories daily. It is when we switch to diet soda that we have reduced our daily calories allowing us to lose the unwanted fat-weight. The problem though, is that we then fail to learn moderation because we can drink lots of diet soda without the calorie penalty of a regular sugar soda.

Depending upon your age, you will likely remember a time before diet soda when most people were thin. Statistically, we could then propose that diet soda has made us fat. But that would not be true.

Pay attention to people's shopping carts in the store at the checkout line and you will see some very heavy people purchasing multiple cases of diet soda, thus proving that diet soda is obviously not the solution to our fat-weight problem.

Doing the right things wrong, can have the reverse effect of what we are trying to achieve. Take care when dieting in order to make sure to do it all right.

There is one big additional problem with diet soda which is little known and seldom mentioned. The problem is that it's true that the theoretical calorie level is substantially reduced in these diet drinks, but the way the body handles the diet drink is an entirely different story. Since the body functions on a chemical basis, the chemistry of some of these diet drinks causes a similar insulin response as that of regular sodas which causes your body to prepare for energy storage in the form of fat. This makes it very easy for your body to store the foods you eat as fat, sometimes even when eating very little. Diet sodas are generally okay to consume, however, if you are unaware of the reality of what they are capable of doing to your hormonal chemistry, then they can be your worst enemy regarding fat weight loss.

Don't Use Food as a Weapon Against Yourself

Always remember that your choice for joy or for early death is your choice alone. Too much of a good thing is usually a bad thing. Overindulging ourselves typically results in self-destruction. With all of the damage that habitual overindulging in food can do, our joy can become our nightmare and cause untold misery for ourselves and for those around us.

All of the diseases discussed in a previous chapter can be yours for the price of overindulgence. And with it you receive the simple luxury of severe discomfort of arthritis, back problems, cancer, artery disease, diabetes, gall stones, acid reflux, kidney problems, liver problems, pancreas problems, sleep apnea, and even a stroke or heart attack and more can all be yours for the low price of ***gluttony***. Don't let the joy of food become a weapon against yourself. *Do all things in **moderation***.

Don't Use Food as a Comfort Item

One of the easiest and most common ways to gain weight is when we use foods as a source of comfort. This occurs because of stress, frustration, disappointment, or any other time we feel like we do not have, or have lost, control. When we have feelings of control loss, then food is very comforting because it is one of the few things we can do that ***we*** control that has very little immediate cost but offers us immediate consolation and comfort.

When we are suffering the frustration of the feeling of a loss of control, food gives us back a little bit of control. But in doing so, we lose even more control because we end with losing control of our fat-weight.

Food is truly a gift and a joy, and using it for occasional comfort is not a problem. But habitually using food for comfort on a regular basis is a serious problem and is one of the main reasons we end up getting fat. This is why trying to get our life under control first can make the difference between losing weight and *losing weight **permanently***. Some of this is discussed in the book *Hot Water - Your Perceived Identity - The Life Repair Manual* and in *Red Hot Marriage - Made in Heaven Filled with Passion and Joy.*

Need for Fat

Here is where the DreamThin concept might see some incompatibility with some members of the medical and the diet industries. The bodies of all humans function the same, but our metabolism rate will vary according to our eating habits, our activity levels, and our muscle mass.

The erred belief that there are born-in metabolic differences from person to person is really mostly due to eating habits, chosen foods, personal daily physical activity levels, and our muscle mass. What we consume, the way in which we consume our calories, and the way we move when we walk, run, get up, sit down and whether we fidget a lot, all have a profound impact on whether or not we will lose or gain fat-weight. These differences in our habits show up as differing metabolic rates. When we are near or at our calorie threshold level, tiny little differences in the way we move can add up to a lot of extra calories burned throughout the course of a day. This is just one of the unknown secrets of people who are "naturally thin".

No foods are particularly bad for us in modest quantities, but no foods are good for us in excess quantities. And while fat in food is often demonized by the food nazis, our bodies need to consume some fat and need to also contain some fat. Fat should be a part of our menu as a rough percentage of our daily eating, just as carbohydrates, proteins, and fiber should be. God has given us an incredible chemical-processing plant in the form of what we call "our body". The body is *designed* to store foods as nutrition and fat that the body will need at a later time for nutrition and energy.

When this God-given system is used properly, it will yield a long happy and healthy life. A problem that has occurred in recent decades with the escalation of the convenience of foods and delicious meals with very high calorie values at a very low price is that this has brought about the many food myths discussed throughout this book.

When we consistently fill our systems with unnecessarily high quantities of food calories, our God-given food-processing-plant-body works precisely as it was designed to work and it assumes that we are in need of storing away extra energy as fat for *future* use. That *future* is now. So, start using that extra energy that is stored as fat-weight until the excess is gone.

Always remember that eating fat does not make us fat, but consuming too many calories of any food energy does make us fat. The fats we consume can be over-indulged in when we abuse them, but in general those fats are a necessity for our body to function properly. Quantity is your key.

Chapter 19

It Starts in Your Head and It Stays There

Weight-loss psychology is critical for all of us to understand. Not the deeper details of weight-loss psychology or the psychology profession, but rather the fact that weight-loss psychology exists and affects us all in a very big way.

When we have wrong ideas about how much we should weigh, or if we believe that we have some sort of genetic disorder, or if we believe that we get fat from eating fat, it all affects our ability to truly deal with the problem. To add to our misperceptions about these and many other issues connected to fat-weight loss, we tend to want to believe these points of incorrect thinking because doing so excuses our current chosen bad eating behavior.

Accepting the Brutal Facts

Facts are facts, and science is science, and unless we face the facts we won't ever permanently lose our fat-weight. Our propensity to taking the easy mental route does nothing for us except to expedite the inevitable increase of our waistline.

Honesty

Brutal honesty is a key element of DreamThin. Tracking our calories and recording them as if they are cents and dollars serves a great purpose in keeping us honest and accurate because dollars and cents are much more relatable and help us to see where we error in our daily eating habits. Doing so will quickly demonstrate to you where that excess unhealthy fat-weight came from in the first place.

With a fairly high amount of accuracy, if you're honest with your recording of your DreamThin Dollars, you will be able to know just how long it will take you to lose the unhealthy excess fat-weight you seek to free yourself from by repaying Fat & Co.

I Can't Do It

It is the frustrations of life and the frustrations of weight loss discussed in this book that discourage our valiant efforts to defeat the fat-weight. When we allow ourselves to think, “I can’t do it”, then we forfeit all of our previous efforts. This is why understanding fat-weight loss and using DreamThin Averaging for your daily tracking are so very important. Eliminating those nasty water retention and bloating spikes through DreamThin Averaging assists a great deal in avoiding those depressing moments that make us feel like we have failed even though we really have not.

When we believe that we can’t, then we don’t even try, which produces only failure for us. You can do it, and you must never say “I can’t” when you know you should say “I can!” Victory is yours when you choose it! Choose victory today, and then next year at this time you will be very pleased with yourself because you will be many pounds lighter. If you fail to do it now, then when this time next year comes along, you will look back and say, "If only I had done it then, I would be finished now!"

Don't Allow Other People to Crush Your Dreams

Don't allow other people to crush your dreams and goals through their petty criticisms. This problem has gotten much worse ever since the dawn of social media. Now every moron with a smartphone can vomit their vile opinions to the entire world in a matter of seconds.

If you post anything about losing weight, you are certain to have some idiot post some demeaning, foolish, and mostly untrue drivel back at your social media account.

It seems that no matter what you do today, there will be some idiot online to condemn you the moment you press "send". Ignore these worthless comments because these people get their kicks from being jackasses, and some of them are being paid or have political agendas when doing this.

If you engage them, then get ready for stupid-on-stupid because they can easily be backed into the corner that they crawled out of, and then they get downright ignorant, cruel, or if you are very lucky they will retreat in rare instances and fade away. But beware that when you engage these types, some of them have an army of accompanying idiots who will make it their mission to try to destroy you.

These types have no self-worth because they believe that they themselves are worthless, and in effort to feel better about themselves, they try to destroy others in attempt to make others feel lower than they themselves do. Never buy into their lies. Just ignore people like that whether in person or online, and try to keep clear of them and keep them out of your life. They are poison, allow them to choke themselves with their own poison, by ignoring them, and consider saying a prayer for them that they awaken from their ignorant slumber.

It is Your Life

It's your life and you have to live it your way. But "your way" should never adversely impact other people. Remember that you have to live with whatever you create in your own life and with how that affects others. This includes the behaviors described in the previous section.

When you're working to get fit and have a healthy personal perfect weight, then you'll likely have to ignore lots of advice regarding the way *other people* believe *you* should live and how you should lose weight.

Amongst those bits of advice, you are likely to find people who will worry that you're an idiot and who don't know what a proper weight for you is. They will want you to stop losing weight before you hit your realistic and healthy goal weight, and they somehow think that you're not going to be able to stop and you're going to have your fat-weight quickly go all the way on down to anorexia.

Ignore these unwise bits of advice and follow what you know is right and true about you and your weight. Most of us have seen this happen to friends and family when they begin to actually start looking great. This is especially true if someone who is familiar with us being fat doesn't see us for a while, and then when we are well-along in our efforts, they are shocked by our appearance and make foolish and ignorant comments. Many of us have even done this to others, and if we have done so we should probably apologize.

As long as you are doing it right and doing so in a safe and healthy way, then nothing anyone says about being too thin matters except what a wise physician or nutritionist or qualified trainer says.

Always remember that is it *your* life, not theirs. ***You*** must live it and live with your efforts, or lack of those efforts. They will not live your life for you if you follow their foolish advice and quit or do it wrong. You and you alone must live with your choices as to whose advice you follow. Those who dish out bad advice typically won't ever step up to help when their advice causes you much hurt and trouble.

Understand the fat-weight loss path you are planning to take and why you are planning to take it. Know how it works and why it works. Achieve your goals for ***you***, and be proud when you achieve those goals. Share your success story to inspire others. It's your life, live it well!

With God as My Witness I'll Never Be Fat Again

Make an Oath to yourself that you will never be fat again and be accurate about your personal perfect target weight. Dedicate yourself to your effort and don't let others talk you into veering from your healthy plotted course. Dreaming thin is really only a description of how weight loss *actually* works. Understand that and adhere to our natural human *design* and you will never be fat again.

Getting a True View of a Week's Portions

Here is a challenge for you to get a graphic grasp on a week of your own food consumption. Every time you eat something during an entire week, take a second one or a second helping and put it in a container shorting nothing in that container. Then at the end of a full week take the containers out and a look at it all. Add up the calories and then divide by seven days. If you do this accurately before you begin any diet and are eating as you "normally" do, then you are likely to be very shocked! The pile of food is usually much larger than people expect, and the average daily calorie amount is often humiliating. This personal demonstration should be done before beginning any diet efforts, but should be done after you have honestly calculated your personal perfect weight. You will thank yourself in the future for giving yourself the gifts of reality and honesty!

Chapter 20

An Example

We have become a fat nation with about seventy percent of us being noticeably overweight. Of course, the big-is-beautiful crowd doesn't like this view, but it is true nonetheless—we are an unhealthy people! This was touched on earlier in this book but as an example, watching older movies from the early to mid-nineteen-hundreds gives clear indication of how different people's weight was years ago versus what we currently see.

You might think that they only had thin actors and actresses making those old movies, and this is typically true for the leading characters, but in general, you have to watch the scenes with then extras crowds back then compared to extras crowds in recent movies. This disparity can also be found in the difference with old news reels versus modern news reports.

There is no question when you pay attention to the waistlines of the people in the movies, that it was in the late 1990s that this problem exploded and the percent of overweight people in the movies began to greatly increase.

Hey Fatty

As mentioned earlier, it is unfair to be insulted and then berate someone if they make a comment about you being fat if you are going to feel praised when someone gives you a compliment about weight you lost. Why can't or won't we hear the good with the bad?

It's because the bad, while true, shames us. When we get angry at someone who calls us fat or even alludes to our weight, we attempt to hide our error with tears or with obnoxious behavior as we attack them for noticing the obvious. Often, we won't even allow a helpful, kind, and well-meaning person to bring it up. We are simply doing this in attempt to hide what we know we are doing wrong.

When someone comments on our weight, we typically choose one of a few wrong options. The first option is to withdraw in humiliation, the next is to lash out and attack them for anything to shift the topic at hand, and the last is to embrace our error with the false big-is-beautiful attitude. The course of action is to accept their notification and then change our behavior.

What's In a Mirror

Lashing out at someone in any manner is unfair, to say the least, unless they are cruelly attacking us. But when it is our own self who is being lashed out at by our own self from looking in a mirror at our own self, then we have a real problem that we have to work through and promptly address.

When we look into the mirror and see the fat sagging all over our body, it doesn't make us feel good about ourselves. Matters can be made worse if we have a cheap mirror that has the ability to flex. When you bend a mirror it distorts the reflection to a point where even a small deviation from perfectly flat will make us look thinner or fatter or taller or shorter than what we actually are.

Some people use this to their advantage to make themselves look fat so they have a deterrent to not eat so much. And if those who do this have an otherwise accurate assessment of their actual weight and health, then it's okay. However, an accurate reflection and good self-control are better, because too often we let the mirror dictate our feelings.

If, unknown to us, a mirror is slightly curved we can get a wrong image of ourself, that can play a very big role in how we feel about ourselves and the progress we are trying to make. If a mirror is going to distort your reflection it should probably be a convex mirror that distorts your reflection to a point of obvious distortion. If a cheap semi-flexible mirror is used it can be difficult to detect that it is giving us a distorted view, and that reflected view is usually only slightly widened or narrowed or increased or decreased in height giving us a false impression of ourselves. Most of us have a hard enough time seeing ourselves accurately. Having a mirror that will only enhance our mental distortion is of no help to us, especially when we are unaware or oblivious to the error in our mirror reflection.

Mirrors can be a good deterrent if we use them properly. Some people will put mirrors on the outside or inside of the cupboard door to remind them of their goals. Depending upon your personality and self-image, this can be of great assistance in keeping you aware whenever you go to eat. It's easy to grab a bite here and there from the cupboard or the fridge, but the movement seen in the mirror and the reflection of our face or body is a stark reminder of our goals.

So, what's in a mirror? We are. And we should use mirrors and understand that they can lie as much as our own minds can if we do not have them installed on a perfectly flat surface and understand how they work.

What You See You Will Be

When we see ourselves in the mirror and that mirror is distorted, making us look even heavier than we are, it can be very discouraging. But our mirror is only the tip of that iceberg. It is our *mental* reflection that causes our greatest distorted view, and some mirrors are of no help.

If our *mental* reflection is fat, it means that fat is how we see ourselves regardless of the quality of our mirror. Many people look into the mirror and see the reflection of their saggy fat body, but their mental reflection resembles that of their glory days of being thin, fit, and healthy. With a better self-image like that, we typically have more power over our fat when we finally choose to conquer it. But when our mental reflection is of a person who is fat, then we associate it with failure and typically feel like a failure, which only serves to discourage us. This is why in the book *Strong Family - A Foundation of Rock - The Family Repair Manual* and in *The Science Of God Volume 4 - Day Six - Evolution versus Man - In Our Image* it explains why getting our head right regarding human evolution versus having been uniquely Created is so important.

We all have been Created in the image of God and this gives each and every one of us great value even if the body is over fat-weight. Your true mental reflection is not some fatty standing in front of a mirror; it is a perfect person Created in the image of God. When we embrace the mental image of being Created in the image of God, it helps us to conquer the visual reflection we see in the mirror and thus helps to get our fat-weight under control.

Always realize that you have been Created "in the image of" and see yourself not as the body you dwell within, but rather as the perfect soul you were Created as. The body is only a temporary home for us and when we understand that our body is not actually us, then it is easier to understand that it is a machine that we are caring for and that we have full control over.

What is a Calorie

Food does not contain calories. Food contains food, and food is ultimately stored solar energy. When we burn that energy, we measure the energy in calories. When dried food burns it produces heat and that heat is measured in degrees Celsius or Fahrenheit. The amount of energy used to heat up and raise one gram of water one degree Celsius at one atmosphere of pressure is called a "calorie".

When discussing fat-weight loss, we are really discussing kilo-calories, or Kcals which is one thousand small calories. But we affectionately call "Kcals" good ol' "calories" because it is easier to say and calculate because we have to deal with fewer zeros. Imagine if a candy bar nutrition label said the bar has two hundred forty thousand calories. It'd probably freak us out a bit.

We don't actually burn calories, we "burn" fat and the amount of energy expended is measured in calories. The idea of "burning" calories is not really accurate, but it is a good way to convey the idea of what we want. The burning perspective likely comes from the fact that it is the burning of food that is done to test its energy content.

As blood circulates through the body, it carries various hormones and when the blood passes by the adjacent fat the hormones cause either the storage of or release of the energy in the fat. As the fat is released due to the signal from the hormones, the fat is carried through the blood and distributed to the needed areas and is used by the muscles in those areas, and then what is not used is ultimately stored as fat or expelled as waste.

The Important Math

There are a few mathematical and scientific facts that dictate all figures surrounding fat-weight loss. The first is that body fat is approximately 3500 calories per pound. This can vary slightly because there are things like moisture content and other micro factors to consider, but the general rule of thumb using 3500 calories per pound has served us well for many years.

Another important math figure is an accurate assessment of your personal perfect weight. When we have this number far off from where it should be, it can be dangerous when it is unrealistically low, and it can be very defeating when it is unrealistically high. It is a number that we should all understand about ourselves whether or not we ever choose to accomplish it. Knowing your personal perfect weight and facing it, has great long-term value.

The other important math is the understanding of the activity or exercise cost of calories consumed. When we realize the approximate calorie cost of something as simple as a single chocolate-covered peanut and the amount of exercise we must do to expend that many calories of energy, it is very beneficial to our fat-weight loss efforts. This understanding also helps us to meter ourselves and know when to say "no" to ourselves when finger foods sit on the table during the holidays and other special occasions.

A single chocolate covered nut can be between ten and thirty calories depending upon the thickness of the chocolate and the size of the nut. A single peanut m&m is about ten calories and is worth about two minutes of jogging. Unfortunately for our desirous-palate, the body is a wonderfully efficient machine that makes a handful of ten chocolate covered peanuts cost in excess of twenty minutes worth of jogging to counterbalance the chocolates.

Knowing and understanding these basics can help to quickly calculate the real fat-weight costs to us every time we take an unnecessary bite.

A Kitchen Survey

Surveys have been made to see what food people typically have on their countertops and if there is any correlation of the foods in conjunction with the people's weight. People who have food or soda at the ready on the counter are as high as thirty pounds heavier than those who don't have food in ready sight on the counter. While a connection appears to exist, we still have to question if the food being out on the counter made them heavier, or if the fact that they tend to snack more often causes a food item to be left on the counter top.

The truth is that it is probably a little of both, because if we don't resist grabbing a snack and we leave that package on the counter, then the next time we pass by it we are far more likely to grab a couple of those chips, or even a small handful of cereal from the box.

Out-of-site-out-of-mind is a good rule of thumb, and if we break down and go to the cupboard to grab a snack, it is important to our fat-weight loss effort to put it away and out of sight when done.

Sorting Out Too Much Information

We all need to recognize the inaccuracies in modern life that are largely due to the abundance of incorrect information often found online. The U.S. Government is rightly bringing to the attention of the public the dangers of being overweight and the epidemic of obesity that has been sweeping the nation for far too long. A big part of the problem is in today's ease of acquiring food and the lower activity requirements needed to do many of today's jobs–things have changed over the years!

Quite clearly, the calorie needs of most individuals have dropped since the computer revolution. We are far more sedentary during the workday than we were several decades ago. Additionally, how much we eat of each food and the ease of acquiring those foods has changed. But for many of us, our knowledge and understand has been unchanged, or even worse, it has been distorted by improper information.

The FDA has chosen to use an easy-to-calculate index of about 2,000 calories for a daily diet to be shown on nutrition labels. But that figure is only a rough index and does not specifically apply to us individually.

We are told what to eat, how to eat, when to eat, and how many calories to take in. But the most important thing to understand when wading through all of this weight-loss noise is what our personal perfect weight should be and how many calories we personally can consume in a day and still lose weight while sleeping as we dream ourselves thin.

There have been no changes in human biology that have affected our weight over the past several decades and there have been no changes in our DNA. But our entire society now has ready access to snacks and hot foods twenty-four hours a day in addition to the sedentary nature of many of our modern jobs.

When we sort out the information, it is critical for us to get a grasp on which information is important and which information is just weight loss noise.

Chapter 21

It's Not My Fault

Whose fault is it that we're all overweight? Is it the food manufacturers fault? Is it the grocery stores fault? Is it genetics fault? Is it our family's fault? Is it science's fault? Who can we blame for our excess fat-weight?

It's always someone else's fault

Amongst our most prominent problems is that we always try to blame anyone else for our own fat-weight problems. So, is it true? Is it someone else's fault? Yes, but only a little bit. Just because your mother made you clean your plate and gave you adult sized servings as a child, does not mean that you must continue to eat oversized servings today. Yes, Mom's cookies are "to die for," but *one* cookie can be enough. There is no reason to eat the entire full plate of cookies.

Us Against Them

What responsibility do those "evil" corporations have regarding our fat-weight problems? According to the media and the agenda-driven food nazis, it is all the food corporations' fault. Some cities have even overstepped their authority and have made large soda sizes illegal. And companies have even been forced, through social media smear-campaigns, to remove certain items from their menus. And so much more has been done to penalize food companies because of our own fat-weight problems and our inability to say "No thank you."

Yet, with increasing restrictions regarding our excessive eating habits that in the past were certainly assisted by the convenience of foods and the sizes of those foods, we still are getting fatter and fatter.

It couldn't be our own fault, after all we don't eat too much, we just eat what they serve us. Right? When you go to the drive-through and place your order, and then they ask if you would like a large for the same price–what do ***you*** say?

Don't Go There

When you eat out and you're offered large-size portions, you need to make some strong-willed choices. Some restaurants serve very generous helpings of food on a "regular" size order. In fact, often a single meal at a restaurant will have as many or more calories than any person should eat in a single day. So how do we handle dealing with those huge helpings? If you are like the rest of us, you'll try to eat the whole thing–and regret it later. But you have choices!

The first choice would be to only eat a small part of each item that they served you, and then ask for a container to take the rest home to eat as leftovers over the next couple of days. You also have the choice of ordering a single meal and splitting it with your spouse. Often you can order a single and ask for two plates at no extra cost. Another option would be to *not* visit a place that has huge serving sizes more than a few times per year. And the last choice is simply, don't go there. It is within your control to not go there, or at least select the other more reasonably sized options that they offer.

Eat It All

Just as Mom serving huge helpings to make sure you're eating enough as a child can cause you to over-eat, so too do the large servings at the restaurants. But you don't have to eat it all. At some point we all have to grow up and take control of our own health. Having a good health insurance policy will not help you lose weight, but saying "no" to extra helpings and upsized meals will.

Our bodies all have a custom daily calorie burn that is based upon our daily activity levels, our muscle mass, and the foods that we choose to eat. If our calories consumed exceeds our total daily calories burned, then *we **will** gain fat-weight*, and can you guess whose fault that is?

Imagine if you went to visit a friend's house and they asked if you wanted a soda. So, you answer "Yes", and when they come back they hand you a 4-ounce Dixie Cup only three-fourths full with diet cola. What would your reaction be? Even if you kept quiet, you would likely be thinking "What the heck?" We are accustomed to large-size portions in our drinks and with our foods.

Just because the restaurant offers you a large for the same price as a small and with free refills, does not mean that you should or must accept that offer. Just because you can buy a one-pound bag of candy for only fifty cents more than the standard single serving size you might grab while standing in line at the checkout, doesn't mean you should. You need to think of those offers as *tests* of your willpower and just say "No."

All eating is our fault. Yes, the food suppliers want to sell us more product, and as competition increases, those packages do tend to get larger and less expensive. But it is you and only you who places that food into your mouth, and *that* is where the food buck stops.

Chapter 22

Question It

You'll notice if you take the time to observe people when discussing fat-weight issues, that most people don't question the facts and figures. And often when we actually do choose to finally ask some serious questions, we often only ask questions that will feed our desire to avoid our problem, thus allowing us to place the blame onto someone else.

How do you ask a question?

Regarding fat-weight loss, questions are usually difficult for us to form in such a way that we can properly ask them or look them up. Because we feel shame, due to our excess fat-weight, we avoid asking questions that we know will place the blame or responsibility on ourselves. When we do this, we are no longer able to drill down to the truth about our situation.

You Must Allow Yourself to Ask

When we try to protect our fragile emotions, we trap ourselves in our lies, and in doing so we get nowhere very fast regarding our weight loss. But when we allow ourselves to ask the tough questions, then we can truly begin to learn. There is much to know when you dig into the deeper details of our biology and fat-weight loss, but we covered the most important aspects in this book.

Ask Yourself How

Other than following the fundamentals of fat-weight loss, you should consider asking yourself how it really happened to you. Look back into your life and figure out when you began to become overweight. For some people it was throughout their entire lifetime. For others, it was when they finished school and were no longer active. For some it was when they got a promotion at work and went from a warehouse job to a desk job. Many moms find it difficult to rid themselves of the unwanted fat-weight after pregnancy.

To begin to understand *how*, we first need to understand *when* it began. With that time pinpointed, you will be able to begin to see the circumstances that caused your waistline to increase. So now that you grasp the circumstances, you must ask yourself "why?"

Ask Yourself Why

When you understand the point at which your fat-weight loss problem began, you can then zero in on *how* it occurred, but that still leaves you asking *why* it occurred. Was it the extra donut at the office that you should not have eaten every single day? Or was eating a safe-place for you when you were frustrated at work, or with the children while trying to keep up with their three-year-old shenanigans? Or could it have been that three or four hundred calorie latte you insist on having every day?

Take the time to really think through these things and get to the core of the *why*. The *why* part is usually somewhat psychological. Not in the sense that you are some sort of nut-case, but rather that maybe it is, or was, stress. Or possibly, that you were simply oblivious and didn't really pay attention until things got really bad with your weight. For many people, it's from very deep pain from emotional injury from when they were younger, sometimes even back to their childhood. And no matter why it occurred, the fact that we are over fat-weight only adds to the psychological aspects.

There is no need to get angry or feel humiliated about any of this. Rather, just make the changes now so that the rest of your life can be as you might have dreamt it to be for all of those years.

Chapter 23

A Matter of Choice

Getting a bit too fat is a matter of choice, but it tends to sneak up on us. When we are young and growing, we play a lot and are very active. Our growing bodies require more energy to grow, so between our growth and our extra physical activity from playing, we are able to eat far more food relative to our size than an adult can, and still not gain excessive fat weight. This is especially true during the teen growth years.

But things have been changing. What was once children skipping rope, or playing hopscotch, or playing ball is now children moving only their thumbs to conquer the most recent game on their smartphone, or texting to friends. The obsession we have with technology is literally killing us.

Surviving the Family Years

Nearly every parent understands how easy it is to gain weight while raising children. As a family we often watch movies together, and to make it an enjoyable experience we typically will have treats while doing so. For many people this is one of the joys of family life, along with just being together. But as parents who often have desk jobs, not only can this add to our joy, it can also add to our waistline. Most of us gain weight during this time of life, but the key is to limit that weight gain. Before you know it, the children leave home and we are left with our unwanted fat. If we have been somewhat careful during these years, then we can get our fat-weight under control in less than a year.

It's good to have these times with our children, but things should be measured a bit because these are *their* formative years. The habits you create for them here will typically last a very long time. People sometimes misunderstand this as to not have any snacks, but this is not what is being conveyed here. Rather, teach them moderation through the serving size they see *you* eat and that *you* serve to them. This way your entire family can survive the family years, and not really gain much if any fat-weight at all.

The Cost of Beauty

Beauty is certainly in the eye of the beholder, but there are fairly clear beauty indicators that dictate our perception of beauty world round. The idea of "beauty" is mostly associated with women and nature, but in truth it applies to everyone and pretty much everything in the right context.

All people have the potential to be beautiful internally, which is up to each one of us, but when it comes to our fatness, beauty is relegated only to the physically visual. This is what the big-is-beautiful mantra is borne of. Just because we are fat does not mean that we are a horrible person inside. While it is true that the outside often reflects the inside, the outside is not a reflection of the person, but rather usually reflects attitudes or troubles we internalize.

So, while big-is-beautiful is not a particularly healthy approach, it must be said that big people are beautiful people and so are thin people, any notion otherwise is a lie. Remember that our body is nothing more than the home of our God-given soul, and the body truly has nothing to do with us being who we are or how beautiful we are as a person.

For some unknown reason, we wrongly associate our fat with our real value and we tend to judge the beauty of the person on the shape of their body. This is unfair prejudice and it has damaged the souls of many of us through the years, making us feel unworthy. But no one is unworthy when they choose to live in God's Truth. Believing that we are unworthy is to believe a lie. Our problem is that the costs of beauty don't stop at our overweight bodies.

Depression

Whether we are willing to admit it or not, being fat typically depresses us and makes us feel like failures even when we buy into the "big is beautiful" lie. When we try to lose weight and can't seem to make any progress, then every bite of that extra cookie makes us feel guiltier and devalues our self-worth. The worst part is when we feel like we have failed ourselves we tend to eat even more food to give us comfort. This is when we must force ourselves to be strong no matter what mistakes we may have made. The reward of success is more than being thin and fit, it is also feeling joyful in your heart knowing that **you** control your physical health and weight.

Keep a positive attitude and never let negative feelings about yourself or any mistake you may make push you into feeling depressed. Every mistake we make can be corrected if we simply try, and then we can use that mistake as a learning experience to know and understand what to avoid in the future.

Female Negativity, But Men Do It Too

It's bad enough that we feel bad when we are over fat-weight, but what about when we are in near perfect shape? We somehow tend to imagine that thin, fit people feel inside the way they look outside, but this is not always true. There are many very beautiful and fit women who feel inadequate even though they have what most other women so desperately want, which is to say, external beauty.

Women are not alone in this, men partake in this type of negativity too, but nowhere is it more prevalent than in the female world. There are certainly some models that have an unhealthily low weight. But the majority of these modeling beauties are well-kept and are very diligent in caring for themselves. After all, they make *millions* for being in great shape.

Sometimes women who feel that they're not good enough and have a poor self-image and are jealous, will comment on the beauties of the modeling world and say that the models are "too thin" or will make some other derogatory comment about them.

The truth is that if most women cared for themselves as well as these models do, then they too could appear to others and themselves as just as beautiful on the outside. And we can assume that if someone was going to pay *you* millions to be fit, that you would most likely be very motivated to do so very quickly. There are few women in this world that are considered so unattractive that they cannot be made to look beautiful in the eyes of society. The rare few who have not been blessed with a face that will be attractive to the entire world are attractive to someone and are often more beautiful inside than many of these models, and typically they have other beautiful attributes as well.

Don't allow other people's negativity or your own negativity to dictate your life. As a human Created in the Image of the Creator, we have no reason to feel negative about ourselves. Put a smile on your face and a skip in your step regardless of being over fat-weight. A great attitude is one of the keys to dreaming yourself thin. When we come to the full realization of our own Creation, then it is easy to hold ourselves in high regard. Never let your current body fat-weight make you feel negatively about yourself. *You* are not your body, you only live there.

Who Are My Friends and Who Are My Enemies?

What is a *friend* and what is an *enemy*? A friend is someone who will stand beside us in times of trouble and who will be honest with us when we are lying to ourselves or are doing wrong. A true friend loves us enough to pull us aside and speak truth to us.

An enemy has the intent to devalue or destroy us. Sometimes these enemies pose as friends, and we might have known them our entire life. But if their words and actions are meant to harm, then they are, by definition, our "enemy". Be careful with the "friends" you keep, because if they are not true friends, then they may devalue you even if they are not intending to. Yet we must be fair about assessing their intent. Just because *we* feel badly because of something they said to us, does not mean that they are an enemy to us. To judge this, you must be honest with yourself in assessing if what they said is true, and if they said it in a reasonable manner when considering our own behavior that caused them to speak up to begin with.

An enemy-friend will say things in such a way as to hurt you with no redeeming or helpful value in their words or actions towards you.

We also have to realize that *we* ourselves could be the enemy-friend to others. Each and every one of us has the same ability to help or harm our fellow man. If we speak ill of others or if others speak ill of us, we must realize that others may speak ill of us and we may very well be speaking ill of others, and all while possibly not realizing that we are doing this. ***We*** can be someone else's nightmare without realizing it.

Accept It and Speak It

Once we have determined our true perfect personal weight and understand the basic elements of dreaming ourselves thin, we need to accept it all and speak our intentions.

We often think that if we share our fat-weight loss goal with friends and family that it will help us to keep those goals. This typically fails because when we don't meet our goals, then we feel even more humiliation and shame.

There's nothing wrong with speaking it to others, but what we miss is to speak it to ourselves. First, we must accept the facts of fat-weight loss discussed in this book, and then we must speak it to ourselves. We all plan to lose weight and we attempt to do so and will go so far as to convince friends and family that we are going to do it, but we fail to convince ourselves. Instead we try to commit ourselves by sharing with others while thinking "This will hold me to my promise." But what we really need to do is to convince ourselves that it is not only possible for us to achieve our personal perfect weight, it is probable when we have full understanding of the DreamThin concept. Don't diet–DreamThin.

Understand and accept the fat loss truths and speak them to yourself and do so with determination and convince *yourself*. And then implement those truths into your life and you are likely to see the progress for which you have been waiting for so long.

Chapter 24

Your Promise of Success

After we accept and speak the truths to ourselves and truly convince ourselves that we ***can*** accomplish our personal perfect weight, then we must make a solemn promise to ourselves that we will stand by these truths and carry them out to fully accomplish our healthy goals.

Why Lose Weight?

It is best if we lose weight for ourselves, rather than to please others. It certainly doesn't hurt to have others in mind, but that dependency is typically not a good idea if it is the only reason we lose the weight.

When we put our weight on their shoulders, then they control it and if we at some point are frustrated with them, it can have profound effects on our state of mind and on our fat-weight. But when we lose fat-weight to please ourselves and for our own health, then only *we* can affect our weight.

We should lose weight for ourselves and for our own health above all, and a part of that should be so that we are here to enjoy our families for a long time so that we can teach them good life lessons. There is really no down-side to achieving your healthy personal perfect weight. ***You*** are the reason to lose the fat.

Put It All On the Table and Be Honest

Look into your past and be honest with your assessment of how you became over fat-weight. When we put it all out on the table for ourselves to see, it is far easier to be honest about our past habits. When we hide or ignore our past it is easier to lie to ourselves and make foolish assumptions that there is something wrong with our body.

When assessing our past, it is impossible to be accurate going forward if we leave things hidden. So, if we have the secret habit of always having a hidden candy bar *and we don't include that in the assessment of our past*, then we will almost certainly do the same in our future. Take the time to write these things down so that they are all on the table at the same time. We need not share this with others, but we do need to understand it all for ourselves.

The importance of dredging up our past habits and putting them on the table, all at the same time, serves to give us an accurate overview of our overall habits. If we fail to do so, it's like when you have a limited budget and fail to list all of your bills when planning what to pay. If the entire list is not well laid out, then we often have a difficult time seeing it all at once, thus causing us to miscalculate our needs and ending with us thinking we have more extra cash than we actually do. It is very easy to forget items when we attempt to do these things by memory alone.

Getting It Right

After you have your past habits laid bare, you can then make proper assessments of those past habits and choose your path to your future and to your goals. When we get it right, it is far easier to achieve those goals. Know your personal facts and figures and understand them. Have a clear grasp of your personal perfect weight and understand it so that you are able to properly explain it to yourself and to others if the need arises.

It is a common occurrence that we believe something but are unable to explain specifically why or what rationale we are using to arrive at that belief. We see this with scientific beliefs and religious beliefs as pointed out in the *The Science Of God* book series and in *Bending The Ruler - Time Travel, The speed of Light, Gravity, and The Big Bang*, but it is also true for our own weight loss. The point is that if we can't fully and properly explain it, then we obviously don't understand it.

We can't really get it right if we don't understand it, unless we're very lucky. First, *understand* what you think you know, and then you might actually "know" it. You *understanding* it and then *knowing* it are the beginning of making it permanent!

Making It Permanent

The ultimate goal in fat-weight loss is not getting to our target weight. Many of us have done that multiple times, or at least we have come close multiple times. The ultimate goal in fat-weight loss is making it *permanent*. Losing the fat-weight is really the easy part of being fit by meeting our personal perfect weight. It is the other part, that pesky *keeping it off* part, that challenges us, and often that is where we fail.

To lose the fat, we simply make sure that we use more calories each day than we consume, and then in a calculable period of days the unwanted fat will be gone–Easy! Then comes that part where we get to eat more again; however, if we failed to create new habits for ourselves, then we will quickly slip back into gaining several pounds per year, or more.

Permanent weight loss is about creating habits that will maintain your weight at a healthy personal level for the rest of your long healthy life. When we understand how the facts and figures work, then we are able to gain a few pounds and quickly lose it again. But if we let it sneak up on us and keep upsizing our clothing, then we will be right back to our fat self within a few years, if not sooner.

Let your clothing be your indicator to your need to reduce your fat-weight. If you are a fully grown adult and your clothes have been fitting well for the past several years, then there is nothing that will change that other than increased body fat.

If you are in your teens, then clothing-fit can still change because our bodies still do some growing during those years. But when we are in our mid-twenties or later, any such changes are minimal and typically take many years. Physical changes later in life are usually not so extreme so as to force us into new clothing, which is why clothing becoming tighter-fitting, is a good aid in reminding us that it's time to take action regarding losing fat-weight. There are very few exceptions to this rule.

Don't buy larger clothing. Instead, lose the fat and reward yourself with new clothing of the same size, rather than giving into the fat and upsizing your clothing. You will never regret staying at a healthy personal perfect fat-weight.

It's All About Balance

When we adjust our habits, it is best that the dominant part of the changes are to our eating. When we create a calorie deficit for the body through exercise alone, then if we ever decide to reduce or stop our exercising, the fat-weight will quickly return.

Calorie reduction is the best means to stay thin. The exercising should be done for the purpose of maintaining and building muscle. We want our body fat level to be dependent upon our eating. It's great to use exercise to assist in losing the fat, but *good eating habits are the only thing* that will *keep* you at your long-term healthy personal perfect weight.

The DreamThin concept is about balance in your eating habits and finding what works best for your life's schedule. Eliminating or greatly reducing our calories before we go to sleep for the night, makes losing weight effortless. Yes, effortless! All we have to do is *nothing* and then go to bed and the weight will slowly come off all on its own. And as long as we don't sabotage our weight during daytime hours we will succeed!

Find your own balance to your own eating habits and eat whatever you want whenever you want, just not as much as you want, and make sure to get all of your required daily nutrients and also make sure you have a reasonable amount time during which your body is forced to burn some fat every single day—nighttime is typically best. Some people choose to do this during the daytime when they are active, but nighttime is typically easier for most of us. It doesn't matter how you do it, but the single DreamThin truth is that we must have a period or periods during the 24-hour day that our body is forced to use calories from our fat system. The calories used during that time must be greater than the calories absorbed during that time.

When you find your personal balance in your eating habits, you can be assured that if your numbers are honest then your fat will reliably disappear and it will stay gone with your new balanced habits.

Your DreamThin Oath

The DreamThin concept is free and is available to every human being on this planet. DreamThin is here to help us all impress these basic concepts into our hearts and minds. Your DreamThin Oath is not something anyone else can make for you because only you control your own wellbeing.

Your DreamThin Oath is an Oath to yourself stating that you will properly understand and implement the natural DreamThin information and the natural functions of your body to achieve your personal perfect weight. And also, that you will share your success with your friends and family so that you all have long and healthy lives with a very high quality of life all of your years.

With your committed DreamThin Oath, you will feel better and stronger, and you will increase your self-image before losing a single ounce. DreamThin never ends and is working for you always. Your DreamThin Oath to yourself is more than losing weight, it is your true new way of life–plus, you will be free of that excess unwanted fat-weight. Live well!

Feel Better, Feel Younger, Live Longer, and Live Better!

Copy these blank Favorite Foods Pages

My Favorite Foods			
Qty/Wt	**Food Item**	**Calories**	**Fat Co Cost**

My Favorite Foods			
Qty/Wt	Food Item	Calories	Fat Co Cost

Journal Pages

When recording your Fat & Co. debt, you do your calculations similar to those suggested in Chapter 6 Part 1 to determine your Starting Debt to Fat & Co. After you have calculated your Fat & Co. debt, enter it in the first line in your Check Book Journal pages. Then figure out how many calories you realistically use every day without any extra exercise (You can use the chart in Chapter 6 on page 75), and then ***deduct*** that amount from the Fat & Co. bill once every day.

Then everything that goes into your mouth must also be entered into your Check Book Journal and must be added to the amount you owe to Fat & Co.

When you exercise, figure the exercise payment and deduct that amount from your Fat & Co. debt.

As you will see in the example shown in the following Check Book Journal, it is very easy to consume more calories than you are using just from eating breakfast and lunch. In the example our debt to Fat & Co., increased by $2.78 for one day, and the example of that day doesn't even include supper. When recording the additions and deductions from your Fat & Co. debt you will quickly become aware of the heavy cost of choosing to eat too many "large" food items. If an average Male about 5 feet 10 inches tall eats a typical large burger he will owe roughly 390 calories or $3.90 to Fat & Co. But then to offset that calorie debt he would have to jog for about an hour just for that burger. As long as your calories consumed are below your Daily Calories Used you have no need for concern, but when your calories eaten exceeds your Daily Calories Used, then the only way that you are not going to gain weight is to add your Daily Calories Used by adding an activity/exercise routine to your day.

Your increased activity level together with your Daily Calories Used must be equal to or in excess of the total calories consumed for nearly every day. If you eat more than you burn daily you will gain weight. If you eat less than you burn daily you will lose weight. You can guarantee yourself that if you are honest about every aspect of weight loss, and you eat less calories than you burn, then you ***will*** lose weight.

Check Book Journal					
Date	**Time**	**Food Item**	**Fat&Co Cost**	**Exercise Deposit**	**Bal**
Life	Time	Starting Debt to Fat & Co.			$2,275.00
6-1	6am	My Base Daily Cals Used		($12.00)	$2,263.00
6-1	6:30am	1-hour morning jog		($3.90)	$2,259.10
6-1	7am	Egg muffin	$2.90		$2,262.00
6-1	7am	Latte	$2.80		$2,264.80
6-1	7am	Donut	$2.00		$2,266.80
6-1	11am	30-minute walk		($0.92)	$2,265.88
6-1	Noon	Large Burger	$3.90		$2,269.78
6-1	Noon	Large Soda 32oz	$3.20		$2,272.98
6-1	Noon	Medium Fries	$3.80		$2,276.78
6-2	6am	My Base Daily Cals Used		($12.00)	$2,264.78
6-2	6:30am	2-hour morning jog		($7.84)	$2,256.94
6-2	7am	Egg muffin	$2.90		$2,259.84
6-2	7am	12 ounce cola	$1.40		$2,261.24
6-2	11am	30-minute walk		($0.92)	$2,260.32
6-2	Noon	Large Diet Soda 32oz	$0.05		$2,260.37

Make copies of these blank Journal Pages

Check Book Journal					
Date	**Time**	**Food Item**	**Fat&Co Cost**	**Exercise Deposit**	**Bal**

Check Book Journal					
Date	Time	Food Item	Fat&Co Cost	Exercise Deposit	Bal

Begin The Life Corner Stone Series

REBOOT YOUR LIFE

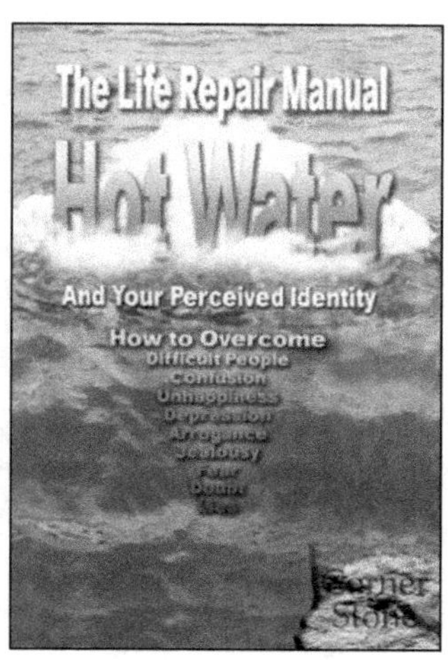

Society forms our perception —You form your identity

We're not stuck... we're trapped by something we can't see. Your True identity is the most powerful thing you own.

Perceived identity is adopted young

It's so familiar—we don't even notice it

It was given—not chosen

Finding your true identity takes some courage and some effort... not everyone is willing to try. Those who do—never look back.

Keep doing the same and nothing changes. Take control today using the right map and find the *you* that you are created to be. Or spend all your hard-earned money in life-long therapy.

Adjust the temperature of your identity and your life... Hot Water is the fresh chapter of life you never knew.

Available wherever books are sold.
Search for:

Hot Water by R Lindemann

Your Life Corner Stones

4 Book Series

Book1

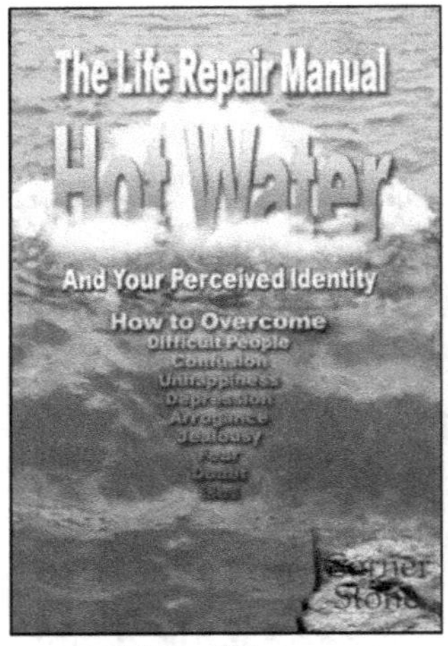

Hot Water

The Life Repair Manual

Book2

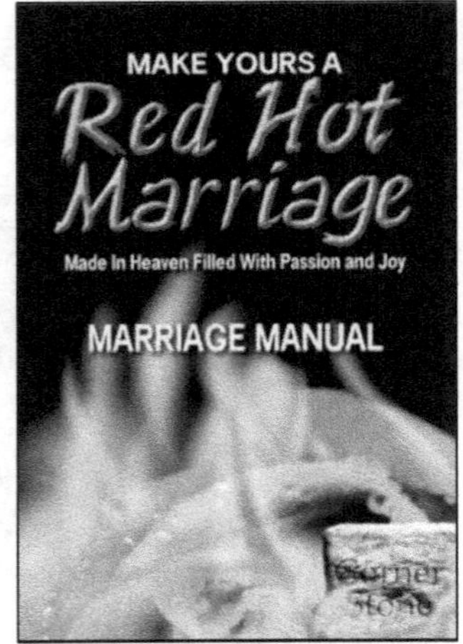

Red Hot Marriage

Made in Heaven

Book3

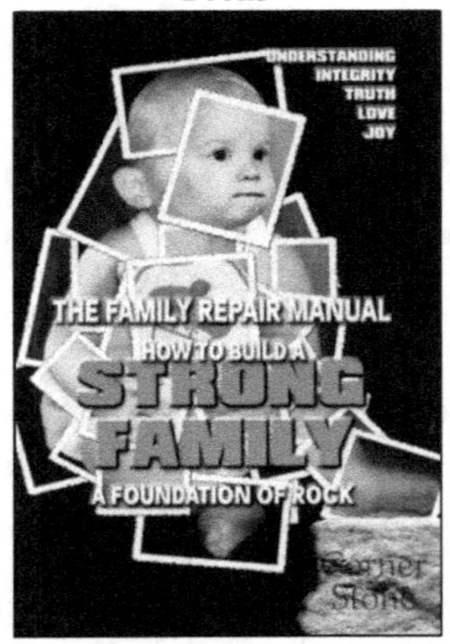

Strong Family

A Foundation of Rock

Book4

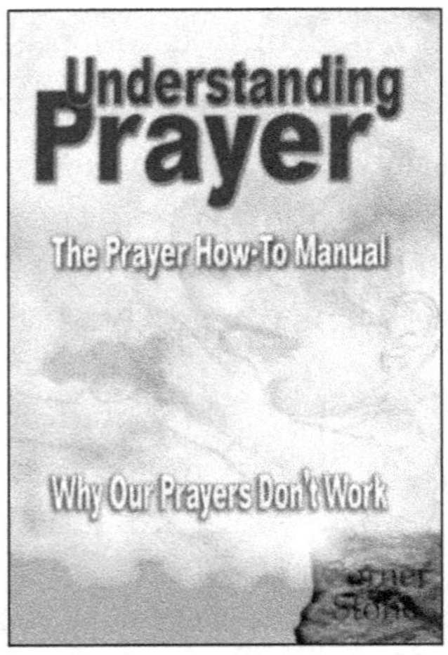

Understanding Prayer

Why Our Prayers Don't Work

Books By R Lindemann

The Life Corner Stone Series

Hot Water – *Your Perceived Identity*
Red Hot Marriage – *Made in Heaven Filled with Passion and Joy*
Strong Family – *A Foundation of Rock*
Understanding Prayer – *Why Our Prayers Don't Work*

The Science Of God Series

The Science of God Vol 1 – *The First Four Days*
The Science of God Vol 2 – *Gravity, Land, Seas, and Evolution of Plants*
The Science of God Vol 3 – *The Creatures – Revolution or Evolution*
The Science of God Vol 4 – *Evolution versus Man – In Our Image*
The Science of God Vol 5 – *Boats, Floods, and Noah – The Deluge*

The Understanding Religion Series

Understanding The Bible – *The Things We Don't See*
Understanding The Church – *Upon This Rock I Will Build My Church*

The Hidden Truth Series

Saint Paul's Controversy – *Saint or Sinner?*
The Truth About Salvation – *What They Won't Tell You*
Understanding Original Sin – *Born Innocent*
Understanding Biblical Law – *The Law is Not Made Void*
Understanding Passover – *Why We Must Observe Passover*

Also by R Lindemann

Dream Thin – *The Weight Loss Repair Manual*
Thank You GOD – *Finding Gratitude in Hard Times*
Bending The Ruler – *Time Travel, The Speed of Light, Gravity, and The Big Bang*

Available wherever books are sold!

Search:

Title **by R Lindemann**

Notes

Notes

Notes

Notes

Notes

Notes

Notes

Notes

Notes

Notes

Notes

Notes

www.ingramcontent.com/pod-product-compliance
Lightning Source LLC
LaVergne TN
LVHW010646110826
845149LV00014B/2968

* 9 7 8 1 9 5 6 8 1 4 2 2 4 *